...rature, though only recently
...al association as an academic
..., ...ave displayed affinities for each other
from their very beginnings. Both disciplines are
founded upon observation and explication of
critical events in human life.

To explore the ramifications of this common
technique and to seek additional interactions
between literature and medicine, the Institute
of Human Values in Medicine brought together
ten individuals—physicians, writers, and literary critics—to talk about present and potential
relationships between literature and medicine.

Joanne Trautmann, who chaired the group,
presents here the texts of the dialogues that
took place in a series of two-day meetings over
a two-year period. The text is recorded in the
form of dialogues enlivened by lyric statements
in prose and poetry. Thus the literary talents of
the participants, as well as their formal knowledge of the healing art of medicine and the
healing powers of literature, are effectively
displayed.

The participants in these dialogues include
Nancy C. Andreasen, perhaps the world's only
M.D./Ph.D. in literature, who has evolved from
critic and composition teacher to psychiatrist
at the University of Iowa College of Medicine.
James C. Cowan, whose wife is a psychiatrist,
edits the *D. H. Lawrence Review* and has written extensively about that author, whose relationship to medicine through *Fantasia of the
Unconscious* and other writings about the
body remain unexplored. Ian R. Lawson received his medical training in Scotland, practicing there and in India before serving as Director
of the Hebrew Home for the Aged and as a faculty member at the University of Connecticut.

Denise Levertov, a nurse in England before
coming to the United States, is a major poet
whose work is closely associated with the late
poet/physician, William Carlos Williams.
Harold Gene Moss is presently on the staff of
the intrinsic merit of wedding these "healing
arts."

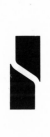

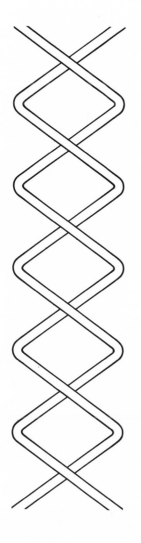

Healing Arts
in Dialogue
Medicine
and Literature

Edited by
JOANNE TRAUTMANN

Southern Illinois University Press
Carbondale and Edwardsville
1981

Published by Southern Illinois University Press in cooperation with the Institute on Human Values in Medicine of the Society for Health and Human Values

This is Report #15 of the Institute on Human Values in Medicine, funded by a grant from the National Endowment for the Humanities.

Feffer and Simons, Inc., London
Manufactured in the United States of America
Designed by Quentin Fiore
Production supervised by Richard Neal

Library of Congress Cataloging in Publication Data

Main entry under title:

Healing arts in dialogue.

(Medical humanities series) (Report of the Institute on Human Values in Medicine; #15)
   Includes bibliographical references and index.
   1. Literature and medicine—Congresses. I. Trautmann, Joanne. II. Series. III. Series: Report of the Institute on Human Values in Medicine; #15.
PN56.M38H4   801'.9   81-8964
ISBN 0-8093-1028-7   AACR2

The great power of art is to transform, renovate,
activate. If there is a relationship between art and
healing it is that.

Denise Levertov
Meeting Five

INSTITUTE ON HUMAN VALUES IN MEDICINE

Contents

Contents

Foreword

Physicians and writers are especially observant of the tragedies and apparent absurdities of human existence. Both groups find their material in death, dying, illness, distress, and other crucial moments of human experience.

But writers and physicians observe for different purposes. Physicians intervene to mitigate or relieve the physical suffering and mental anguish they encounter. They discern, classify, and treat illness. Writers clarify and interpret—thus identifying meaning in events. They may even confront the reader with the meaninglessness of the situation being described. Of the writer's craft, John Henry Cardinal Newman said: "Literature stands related to man as science stands related to nature . . . Literature is to man what autobiography is to the individual. It is his life and remains."[1] Literature is quite simply the autobiography of our species.

Medicine and literature have had affinities for each other for centuries. The facts of medicine are grist for the writer's mill; the writer's evocations of man's fate are stimuli for reflections of thoughtful physicians. A primary source for the physician is the personal history of each patient, which may be thought of as the patient's life story or novel.

The facility for simultaneous detachment from and attachment to life is common to literature and medicine. Indeed, the ability to couple observation and participation provides an opportunity for dialogue between seemingly otherwise disparate disciplines. In order to explore the ramifications of this common methodology and to pursue other possible interactions between literature and medicine, the Institute on Human Values in Medicine initiated a series of meetings placing writers and literary scholars in conversation with physicians. The Institute's ultimate purpose is to examine how literature may contribute to the education of the physician and enable him to gain a better comprehension of the human values with which he deals daily. Under the auspices of the Institute, this dialogue is part of a larger schema designed to examine the intersection of medicine and medical education with history, the visual arts, religion, and the social sciences.[2]

The fruit of discussions between the talented persons invited to participate in a series of two-day meetings over a two-year period is presented in this book. The text is recorded in the form of a dialogue interspersed with lyric statements in prose and poetry. In this way the literary talents of the participants, as well as their more formal knowledge of the healing art of medicine and the healing powers of literature, are combined most effectively.

Joanne Trautmann, who chaired the group, has exquisitely distilled the essence of these meditations and deliberations. The unfolding process whereby these sensitive and creative people came to understand their common problems and air divergent views is fascinating in itself. The dialogue reveals something of the participants' own lives and gives eloquent testimony to the way medicine and literature are unified in their healing intention.

The group was commissioned to ask critical and crucial questions. This it has done brilliantly. Simplistic answers are not, and cannot be, forthcoming. Yet as the dialogue unfolds, the reader perceives more forcefully than a simple exposition might allow how medicine and literature reinforce each other and yet also how they remain—and must remain—distinct enterprises.

For the medical educator the value of teaching literature *pari passu* with medicine should emerge clearly from these pages. By virtue of its capacity for evoking emotions, the study of literature can teach empathy with regard to experiencing illness in ways that the clinical lecturer cannot. Through the artful use of word and phrase, literature teaches something of the nuances of verbal communication and the importance of both clarity and suggestion in the use of language.

A patient's history is a narrative; students can gain some comprehension of what constitutes a proper narrative form by ascertaining the ways in which a writer tells his story. Students can also benefit from an awareness of what it is to *be* a physician through a vicarious experience with the lives of physicians, their families, and their patients in the world's literature.

Finally, literature has its intrinsic worth for the physican as a source of enrichment of life and a diversion from the weighty tasks of everyday. Literature is itself a healing art: healing physician, patient, and writer alike.

It is the hope of the Institute that this book, along with the other published dialogues between medicine and the humanities, will suggest ways to enhance the education of future physicians, to make them more responsive to the awesomeness of the healing relationship.

Edmund D. Pellegrino, M.D.

Acknowledgments

Meeting Two. Reprinted by permission of Farrar, Straus and Giroux, Inc. From "Waking in the Blue" from *Life Studies* by Robert Lowell. Copyright © 1956, 1959 by Robert Lowell.

"The Surgeon as Priest," from Richard Selzer *Mortal Lessons*, is included here by special permission of the publisher, Simon & Schuster.

Permission to quote from the works of D. H. Lawrence by the estate of D. H. Lawrence, the estate of Mrs. Frieda Lawrence Ravagli, and Laurence Pollinger, Ltd., as published in the titles listed below, is gratefully acknowledged.

William Heinemann, Ltd.: *Lady Chatterley's Lover*, 1961

The Viking Press, Inc.: *Etruscan Places*, 1968; Warren Roberts and Harry T. Moore, eds., *Phoenix II: Uncollected, Unpublished, and Other Prose Works by D. H. Lawrence*, 1968; Vivian de Sola Pinto and Warren Roberts, eds., *The Complete Poems of D. H. Lawrence*, 1971

Random House, Inc.: *St. Mawr and The Man Who Died*, 1959

Meeting Three, "Artist to Intellectual (Poet to Explainer)." Denise Levertov, *Life in the Forest*. Copyright © 1978 by Denise Levertov. Reprinted by permission of New Directions.

Participants in this dialogue acknowledge with gratitude Edmund D. Pellegrino and the Board of the Institute on Human Values in Medicine, who first envisioned this project and then provided the support and encouragement necessary for its completion.

The Institute received generous financial assistance for the project from the National Endowment for the Humanities under Grant EH-10973-74-365. The Southern Illinois University Foundation-Medical Humanities Fund provided additional support. We thank the persons in both institutions for their contributions.

Acknowledgments

Special thanks is due to Institute Board members E. A. Vastyan and Mary Stephens, and Institute Director of Programs Thomas K. McElhinney, each of whom contributed valuable time and expertise in ways not readily apparent in this book.

Eileen Thompson deserves thanks for her work as the recorder for the meetings, a difficult job which she managed with skill. Joan Bernardo, June Watson, Helen Melnyk, Margaret Moehle, and Marilyn Flanigan expertly typed the final manuscript.

Prologue: Dramatis Personae

In the spring of 1975 nine people met for the first time at Sugar Loaf Conference Center in Philadelphia. We were humanists: professors of literature, writers, and physicians; and we were committed to meet four times more in the next eighteen months to talk about present and potential relationships between literature and medicine. Our sponsors, the Institute on Human Values in Medicine, told us only to conduct a dialogue about those conceptual matters we deemed of most value or interest or appropriateness to our skills, and to produce, at the end of it all, some written document that could be shared with others who were curious about our subject.

We had a luxurious freedom. But freedom was essential, for the subject of literature and medicine hadn't much of a history to guide our dialogue.[1] We couldn't assign ourselves obvious topics and proceed to cover the field. If that had been possible, what you would have in your hands today would be a far neater document, perhaps nine essays on nine discrete aspects held together with a large staple disguised as an editor's introduction, something we would all recognize as "proceedings" or "transactions." What you have instead is an attempt to let you overhear our discussions: what we said to each other, what satisfied us and worried us, even in one case, because it was relevant, which wine we drank for dinner. To be sure, there are papers in the pages that follow. Each of us wrote out something for one of the meetings. But some of the papers are more scholarly than others; some more like informal essays—musings on personal matters, on art objects, on the issues of the current dialogue, on the nature of human potential itself; some are poems.

Every aspect of this book is intimately connected to the people who are doing the talking. Therefore, in lieu of the conventional notes on contributors, I offer brief sketches of the participants. We were nine, I have said. But that is not quite accurate. We were joined from time to time by two board members from the Institute on Human Values in Medicine—Professors Mary Stephens now of Johns Hopkins University (formerly of Brown) and E. A. Vastyan of The Pennsylvania State University College of Medicine, whose fields are literature and religious studies, respectively—and at every meeting by the Institute's Director of Programs, Thomas McElhinney. There was also a tenth dialogist, who left after one meeting but who remained a shadowy, challenging presence because he had said, on departure, " 'and' is a neutral word. You can link anything and anything else, and pretend for awhile that you have a subject, but do you really have one?"

Those who remained were, in alphabetical order:

Nancy C. Andreasen, who may be the world's only M.D./ Ph.D. in literature. First she was one, an English professor with a special interest in John Donne, and now the other, a psychiatrist at the University of Iowa College of Medicine. She rather distressed us at the first meeting by declaring that one of her professional selves had very little to do with the other. She had, she said, written articles for the medical journals on mentally ill writers, but essentially she was a psychiatrist with literary interests, rather than anyone who could serve as a model of someone whose professional field was literature-and-medicine. Perhaps by the end of the meetings Nancy's interests, if not actually hyphenated, were intellectually intertwined in new ways. In any case, the story of why she had left English for psychiatry (she felt that she could do more good as a doctor than as a literary critic and teacher of freshman composition) and what kind of psychiatry she practiced (rather more scientific and drug-oriented than otherwise) provoked hours of response from the other dialogists, especially from

James C. Cowan, whose wife is a psychiatrist practicing a kind of dynamic therapy of which Jim enthusiastically approves, as he also generally approves of Freud. He was invited to join the dialogue group because of his interest in D. H. Lawrence. At the University of Arkansas, Jim edits the *D. H. Lawrence Review* and has written extensively about that author, whose relationship to medicine through *Fantasia of the Unconscious* and all his writings about the body, really, are still underexplored.

Ian R. Lawson got his medical training in Scotland, practicing there and in India before coming to Hartford, Connecticut, as Director of the Hebrew Home for the Aged and faculty member at the University of Connecticut's medical school. Ian's value to the group derived partly from that multi-national experience, particularly since two of the three countries encourage doctors to see medicine in its social, cultural contexts and don't discourage doctors from being articulate speakers and writers. Ian also had a thorough acquaintance with some of the recent theory about language in medicine and, as an internist, the most direct contact of any dialogist with primary patient care.

Both these facts were of great interest to *Denise Levertov*, who had been a nurse in England before coming to this country and to a major career as a poet. Her literary alliance with William Carlos Williams, the finest American doctor-poet, and her concern that art be involved with life's real battles—notably her role as the prominent poet-pacifist of the Vietnamese War era—made her, predictably, a central member of our group. An unexpected aspect of her participation was her insistence that life's battles need not draw an artist into madness. On this point she agreed with Nancy, brought out what she thought "romantic" or "Romantic" dichotomies in other dialogists, and probably helped to precipitate the group's having to deal with the whole issue of dichotomy.

Harold Gene Moss is currently on the staff of the National Endowment for the Humanities. As a member of both the Departments of English and Community Health at the University of Florida, he had done some serious thinking about literature and medicine before beginning this dialogue. He had once told a group of community physicians, for instance, that from the individual patient's point of view the situation of serious illness was essentially tragic, but from the doctor's sequential point of view, it was comedic. On that occasion Gene enthralled his only literary colleague present, but may have led a few other members of his audience to believe he had said they laughed in the face of death. So when Gene joined our group, he eagerly anticipated talking with a larger group of sympathetic colleagues than he had yet encountered in his area of dual interests.

The history of literature and medicine may be short, but a good deal of it has been written by classically educated physicians, foremost of whom in this country is *William B. Ober*, who for many years has addressed his medical colleagues on subjects such as William Carlos Williams, D. H. Lawrence, and Anton Chekhov, which have also drawn the scholarly attention of other dialogists. Bill is a scientist, a pathologist who knows his work thoroughly and claims he would be bored by it if it were not supplemented by his interest in literature, the arts, and history. He is also a self-proclaimed gadfly and in this role provoked one major conflict and several minor scenes, all of which usefully pushed the group towards resolutions.

Richard Selzer, New Haven surgeon, essayist, and short story writer, came to the dialogue with one book behind him, the second just ahead. He proved generous about sharing his new work with us as he wrote it. What he wrote was good, and everyone participated in the excitement of creative work on Dick's topics—the body in love and illness, the surgeon as celebrant—which were, after all, our topics too. Dick probably came closer than any of us to living out a life concerned equally, and not precisely separately, with literature and with medicine, but others of the dialogue group also lived without the conventional boundaries, including

Elizabeth Sewell, poet, novelist, literary critic, metaphysician, teacher, integrator, magician. After finishing our dialogue, Elizabeth went on to start one with the neurologists interested in the two halves of the brain. Her subject may be, ultimately, the imagination and the capacity of human consciousness. Dismissing one of our skirmishes about mired dichotomies (which was more real, poetry or science? who mad, who not?), Elizabeth announced, "I am mad one hundred percent of the time and sane one hundred percent."

Joanne Trautmann spends most of her time teaching literature to medical students at The Pennsylvania State University

College of Medicine and part of her time editing the *Letters of Virginia Woolf*. Because she admired them all, Jo invited the other eight to join her for the dialogue and then watched like a Steppenwolf to see how they got on together, how they grouped, and regrouped.

*Healing Arts
in Dialogue*

MEETING ONE

Exposition

23 May 1975

DENISE LEVERTOV   In order to speak truthfully, we have to trust, which can't come without laying forth and sharing our feelings, tensions, and expectations.

NANCY ANDREASEN   There was a time in my life when I felt I had made myself unequipped for the world I preferred because I was too literary for the medical people, and, by the time I had spent a couple of years in medicine, too hardheaded for the literary people. Once while I was in medical school, I went to a session composed of people from the English and Psychiatry departments. As they spoke, it became evident to me that the English people didn't understand the things the psychiatrists were talking about. Each group, in fact, was using the same words to mean different things. I came to the conclusion that it is difficult to create a dialogue between literature and medicine.

Why did I switch from literature to medicine? Well, I had my first child and finished my first book at about the same time. In thinking about the delivery, which had been rather complicated, I compared it to the work involved in the writing of my book. When I realized what even one physician accomplished in one individual childbirth, I admitted its superior importance over anything I could do as an English professor. And when I weighed what potentially I could do in medical research against what I had done in literary research, I decided to change my life. For me the choice has been a happy one. I no longer feel discomfort from living in two worlds, even though some of my medical colleagues think of my literary interests as an ornament to attract bright, East Coast residents!

DENISE LEVERTOV   You are speaking with some irony of your colleagues, but it seems to me that *you* describe your literary interests in similar terms.

NANCY ANDREASEN   It goes back to what is personally rewarding for me. Looking at life realistically, I've realized the necessity of having some kind of positive reinforcement and I am much happier now. I see a fair volume of patients, and that in itself is probably the core of my sense of satisfaction. I find seeing patients ultimately much more rewarding than teaching students or writing a book on John Donne. If I were a good creative writer (anybody who does literary criticism would rather be a good writer than a good literary critic), then that might have contented me. I wasn't unambitious.

DICK SELZER   I accept this as a personal statement—what worked for you.

NANCY ANDREASEN   That's all it is.

DICK SELZER   That's all it is, quite obviously. I happened recently to read an essay by Emerson called "The Poet," in which he states that the only true doctor is a poet because the poet observes and interprets, in other words, *diagnoses*, and on rare occasions can even prophesy. I believe that. In your initial statement you did seem to imply that you could do so much more of value as a doctor. Like Denise, I question that conclusion. I think that the poet is singularly gifted with the ability of finding the way to heaven, so to speak, by imparting a vision about all the workaday business of medicine in which you and I are engaged.

NANCY ANDREASEN   I agree wholeheartedly. I just knew that I was not going to be *the* poet. Most of my students were not going to be poets either.

BILL OBER   Well, I've been a doctor a little longer than Nancy, and *I* question the value of practicing medicine. Although I've done so for a number of years and I don't consider myself a poor doctor, I'll be damned if I know if I've done anybody much good. Oh, it is a perfectly legitimate way of spending one's life. It's satisfying, up to a point. But I think I want something more out of life.

DENISE LEVERTOV   What if you save the lives of people who really want to live?

BILL OBER   Well, that's nice. But like Nancy, I'm talking about my personal satisfaction. After you've become an accomplished physician it's not that big a deal—not much different from trying out a new recipe. You want to see if you can make it work. After you've made the recipe a half dozen times, it becomes routine.

DICK SELZER   Now, I cannot let that go!

BILL OBER   Bear in mind that as a surgeon, you are on the firing line directly, and I'm at one remove.

DICK SELZER   You mean because I deal with living tissue and you deal with dead tissue?

BILL OBER   No, those pieces of dead tissue are little pieces of living people.

DICK SELZER   Right. They all pertain to the patient. We are both engaged in what I would like to think is a priestly business; that is, making sick people who want to live, well. I must say that I found your casual, rather charmingly put, but to me shocking assessment of your role unacceptable.

DENISE LEVERTOV   There are two things being discussed here. One is the essential value of what you are doing, and the other is your response to experiencing that value. What seems peculiar, Bill, is that although you don't deny the value of medicine, you don't feel good about contributing to something which you find of value. Why is there that hiatus? Why isn't there a connection between believing something to be of value and getting satisfaction from it?

BILL OBER   Many marriages have foundered on that very rock.

DICK SELZER   There is a peculiar lack of passion here.

THE TENTH DIALOGIST   Bill, would you describe the primary function of pathology as identifying patterns and putting them together? If so, how remote is that function from the primary research mechanism you employ in writing your psychobiographical criticism of literary topics?

BILL OBER   Not at all remote; it's the same thing. It's classifying disease. Finding disease, classifying it and analyzing it. There is no difference.

THE TENTH DIALOGIST   Couldn't you generalize that just a little further and compare the primary function of pathology to finding patterns of relationship not strictly medical?

NANCY ANDREASEN   Bill doesn't get the immediate feedback of his discoveries. But if physicians discover preventive techniques for depression or schizophrenia, feedback comes quickly. I find that as exciting as it can be.

BILL OBER   The feedback I get wouldn't make a rat's nerve twitch.

NANCY ANDREASEN   When I was teaching English, I didn't get much feedback either. I had to teach basic composition, which was a deadly experience. The only courses I enjoyed were honors courses because the students were interested and interesting. With the other kids I was just pounding my head against the wall. Although they could learn some things by rote, getting the concepts across was an entirely different matter.

BILL OBER   We've all had residents like that, too.

DENISE LEVERTOV   What do you do now when you've got a recalcitrant patient?

NANCY ANDREASEN   You do the best you can to make him realize he must take his medicine. That's another thing I've learned about the medical profession. Intelligence is not an important value. It's fun when you have a bright patient, but it's a relief to realize that you don't have to make judgments about people based on IQ.

JO TRAUTMANN   There are so many other questions we need to ask you, Nancy, because you are the only one of us here who has degrees in both literature and medicine. For instance, what do you think in general of psychological or psychiatric interpretations of literature? That's one of the obvious connections between the two fields, and you've done some writing of that sort yourself.

NANCY ANDREASEN   Well, there are a lot of interesting things I can do as a psychiatrist studying literature. However, I still feel that when I write an article such as the one I wrote about Sylvia Plath for the *Journal of the American Medical Association*,[1] I'm compromising literary principles. That is not really a literary article. That is a medical article.

BILL OBER   That's a tailored piece for a specific journal. There is nothing wrong with that.

NANCY ANDREASEN   The other area in which I've combined psychiatry and literature is my work with the nature of the creative process and the extent to which imagination influences it. There seem to be no right words to talk about this process, but it centers around the extent to which creativity is dependent upon a bit of madness in terms of sheer imagination. This in turn brings up the question of whether or not creative people have a genetic constitution which predisposes emotional problems of one sort or another. This is an area in which I've done quantitative research. I've seen that creative people do have a higher rate of mental illness in their families than people who are not.

JO TRAUTMANN   Denise, what expectations did you have for these meetings?

DENISE LEVERTOV   Because of the title for our work, "the healing arts," I felt pretty sure that one of the things that might get talked about was the concept of doing literature as a form of therapy. I want to make my position on that very clear because

I think that they are two different things. I want to distinguish between self-expression and art. Take a look at the word "express" as the nursing mother is said to "express milk." Is that what the function of art is? No, quite the contrary. It has a transformative and absorptive function. It's not a matter of getting rid of feelings but of recognizing them, absorbing them, and transforming them. The more subjective kind of art is really an attempt to get things off one's chest. Certainly this is what happens when people use poetry in mental hospitals, drug rehabilitation programs, prisons, and so forth. I'm not saying this is wrong. It just should be pointed out as wrong when they don't distinguish it from art. People may feel better writing with a pen, but it's not going to produce a work of art because it's more in the nature of a gesture. It's like stamping your foot or jumping up in the air.

Then there were two topics on that list you sent delineating possibilities for discussion in this dialogue[2] to which as a practicing poet I might be able to contribute something. One is concerned with responsibility to self versus responsibility to the community; the other with the nature of objectivity in medicine and literature. I would like to detach the word "objectivity" from the word "cold." I know that cold objectivity is of no use in the arts, and it might be interesting to know whether it is in fact useful in medicine.

BILL OBER   I always associate the word with "clarity."

DENISE LEVERTOV   "Clarity" is also associated with "coldness," though, and all those entanglements need to be untangled. "Clarity" has associations of "tonelessness" and of "right illumination." But clarity is the comprehension of something which is in its nature mysterious. It is not necessarily brought about by shining a bright light on it, but rather by the experiencing of its mystery.

BILL OBER   You know, this is precisely one of the points at which my particular trade comes up. The major portion of my work is done at a microscope with a very clear, reasonably high intensity light coming through an object illuminating its mystery (or what we think is its mystery). To me this is not cold clarity. I hope it's objective, it's illuminating, it's neutral.

ELIZABETH SEWELL My internal tigers are beginning to growl at what is going on [the talk of literature and medicine as two separate disciplines], and I'm in trouble. If I'm too radical for everybody, I shall feed my tigers from time to time, you know, and keep them quiet. But at some stage we should really try to think about unity.

I have a firm conviction that scientists and artists belong together. I was one of the victims of our whole system of education, which splits us so early. I had a marvelous education. It was so good I never questioned it until I was twenty-seven, and then I questioned it with such fury because something very strange happened to me. I was working on my Ph.D. at Cambridge, a very respectable humanist concentrating on late nineteenth-century French poetry. I had a card index this long, had written two chapters poorly, and was getting very depressed.

It was in October of 1946. I have good reason to remember the date because if I had realized what would happen, I don't think I ever would have taken the action I did. I made a whimsical decision, one afternoon, to pretend nobody had ever written about poetry and language and to start thinking about things for myself. Then something simply astonishing happened. I suddenly realized that I had no idea how to think! So I started to try to learn how to think. The experience was most peculiar, very frightening. I saw that thinking had something to do with patterns, with relationships. And yet no one knew about relationships.

One day I was thinking about words and I concluded "They seem to be complex variables." That was a term from higher mathematics. I had hated math all my life, loathed it. But I went down to the library, into the section labeled "Mathematics," and I thought, "I'm going to start!" And right in front of my nose I saw Whitehead and Russell's *Principia Mathematica*. I started there. Of course four-fifths of it I couldn't understand, but one-fifth, I could. And that year I read math and logic; everything in the fields I could lay my hands on. I thought about poetry and language. I wrote nine chapters, and

7

sent the manuscript to my college as my dissertation. I was promptly fired.

I had started to think, but I had thought myself into a whole different framework and have never gone back. So that's why I growl at the rest of you from time to time. I simply don't believe in the split between science and art, or medicine and humanities. I saw the same thing when I began teaching poorly educated blacks in Mississippi. They hadn't had my experience and hadn't, therefore, been split as I was. I knew students who were as good in calculus as they were in poetry, in economics as in painting. So that's one thing that brings me here—I love to be with people who are in science, and to affirm the unity of science and the arts.

The other thing I realize as we talk is that I'm enormously interested in vitality and health, in energy, in the energy that Blake says is eternal delight. I'm interested in it myself because I have só much more than when I was twenty. I want to think about what health is, and to think about this in connection with medicine. I'm here to offer my own life to this process, and to accept whatever of yours you want to give, because it's not just a thinking thing. One's life is one's message.

JO TRAUTMANN I've listened to your story with great interest, Elizabeth, and I've read your books with admiration, but, to get the worst out on the table, let me confess that there are times when I don't want to know about higher mathematics; when I think, "I don't have all the time I need to learn everything about literature, let alone something that may sidetrack me in the short run." I have moods when I think that Art is All. Yet, of course I understand your yearnings for unity and have experienced them, too.

BILL OBER Denise, let me ask you about studying anatomy when you were a nursing student. First permit me a brief digression about the way anatomy is taught. Too much is taught. I expect medical people to know the heart and kidneys are there but it's not necessary to know where every little cutaneous nerve goes. Pathologists do the same thing. We examine all students as if they were all going to be anatomists or pathologists. This isn't necessary.

NANCY ANDREASEN   You mean the time could be freed for the study of literature!

BILL OBER   Dick, do you agree with me?

DICK SELZER   No, I don't. I couldn't disagree more. My view of the study of medicine (what we're talking about seems to have little to do with literature) is that without anatomy the study of medicine is absurd because anatomy is the very body itself, the touchstone, the essence, the whole thing. If you get so utilitarian ("I don't have to know because they never ask me") or so ethereal as to treat medicine as an abstraction and never look at the body, which is really the business district of medicine—

DENISE LEVERTOV   It's like syntax.

DICK SELZER   For me, anatomy was the structure—these gullies and canyons—which attracted me to medicine. It is where my heart is. That is what I write about.

DENISE LEVERTOV   The analogy for me, in my limited experience of studying anatomy and physiology, was that trying to memorize all those muscles was like the way they used to teach languages: teaching the grammar endlessly and never teaching people to speak the language. Grammar divorced from the language. And so anatomy was interesting for me when it was related to how the things actually were—the physiology.

ELIZABETH SEWELL   You know, I really question that. I also wanted to make a statement awhile back about learning math. I think all—I was going to say "children's," but I think all —minds have a passionate affection for, and almost a union with, pattern. I'll bet as a child you looked at patterns in the linoleum.

DENISE LEVERTOV   Oh, yes, I drew.

ELIZABETH SEWELL   There it is—you're a mathematician! And that's how one does grammar. I think of myself learning Latin when I was nine (a language I obviously was never going to speak). Five cases! Ablative—how exciting! Some day I have to learn Russian, where there are ninety-nine cases, or something like that. I adored grammar because it was so patterned.

BILL OBER   I agree with you. I'm very attracted by pattern and structure. And was perfectly happy to learn grammar for its own sweet sake.

DICK SELZER   And I anatomy. The study of anatomy, for some, is not a utilitarian pursuit, but rather a kind of worshiping of perfection, of a highly organized structure. One stands back in awe and marvels.

DENISE LEVERTOV   Well, *I* marveled at how it *moved*.

JO TRAUTMANN   In any case—

THE TENTH DIALOGIST   Why did I come to this meeting? I suppose a good place to start is the assumption that if we have a continuous culture for the next couple of hundred years that human beings as we now think of them are going to be almost totally irrelevant. And I have not yet made up my mind whether I think this matters or not. One of the two or three principal causes of the end of what we now mean by human beings is Western medicine. Therefore, I have a keen interest in what Western medicine is doing. It seems that until recently people in medicine have been doing it without realizing what's being done. This practice has changed in the last five years or so. But I still find that most undergraduates planning to go to medical school either are not examining it (they're too busy taking biochemistry), or they in effect say, "This is why I want to be an undergraduate at a liberal arts college—so that I can think about it now, but I know I must put it away for life once I get launched on a career." It seems as if the only people who *have* thought about these matters are a few philosophers and a lot of science fiction writers. I don't feel comfortable with the word "humanist." I'm not as good at perceiving patterns as some of the people here. I can't identify the class to which people who think about these things belong.

To expand a bit: however much mystery and beauty there may be in the human body, Dick, it does seem to have a lot of breakdowns. There are much better designs, I understand, that can be made for an organism that would be capable of synaptic connections. To me it seems clear that organ transplants and genetic research are only the tiniest beginning. Arthur Clarke in *Profiles of the Future*[3] guesses that about the year 2090 there will be a good working model for a mechanical body to handle the human brain, to receive more than different kinds of sense impressions, and to be free of headaches, arthritis and most forms of wearing out. I don't want to see this happen, but I can't make up my mind whether or not that's a mere clinging to some kind of transition stage.

BILL OBER   Thank God, I'll be dead by then.

JIM COWAN   I'd like to get into this discussion by responding to several matters that have been raised today. To begin with, when I was invited to join this group, I wondered as Nancy did what possible links there could be between literature and medicine. I thought immediately of some research topics: for instance, literature about certain medical syndromes—there's *The Magic Mountain*—and *Camille*. Or we could concentrate on authors with certain illnesses as in psychobiography, etc. One could also write about doctors in literature (who are often treated uncomplimentarily in the twentieth century, by the way), such as the two in Virginia Woolf's *Mrs. Dalloway*. All of these topics are possibilities. Yet none of them, it now seems to me, quite hit the mark of what is needed for medical education.

I also had some preconceptions about members of the dialogue group, but these have not lasted. I felt I had reasons for identifying strongly with some persons because of the backgrounds they bring to the dialogue and not particularly identifying with others. Intellectually, the person I most expected to identify with was you, Nancy, but I don't. Whereas someone like you, Dick, I would not have expected to have much in common with since I know nothing whatsoever about surgery and don't feel particularly attracted to it as a field. And yet the ideas—and more importantly, the attitudes and feelings—which you expressed about the body, the flesh, its wonder and mystery are something that I can very strongly agree with and admire. I have often encountered these ideas in works of D. H. Lawrence, but not at all from the same position.

Key words seem to linger in my mind. For instance, we have emphasized the importance of the words "process" and "unity." We've talked of the "wonders of the body," almost as if they made up a work of art. If literature could help medical students realize the importance of process, unity, and physical wonder, then it has a useful function.

We've all read about the Nazi doctors who were technically proficient but who performed terrible experiments on human subjects. I remember reading in a Bruno Bettelheim book about an obstetrician who did a perfectly sterile delivery, and then sent both mother and newborn baby to the gas chamber.[4]

I'm not sure that literature teaches morality. Perhaps the average literature scholar would have done the same thing as that doctor, or worse. Much of scholarship in literature is very dehumanizing and doesn't contribute at all to the humanities. Some of our technical proficiency might have led us to the same kind of acts. But I certainly think that anything that can help a medical student relate to his own body and to other persons as humans, rather than solely as objects, can be beneficial. Can literature do this? If literature can encourage students to be aware of "process" in other people, of the "wonder" of other people's bodies, and consequently of them as something holy, then literature can be valuable.

I have no magic formula for accomplishing these goals, but because to me literature is the most all-inclusive discipline, it can bring home to students some awareness of the "unity" we were talking about. If it can help them to become humans treating others as humans, rather than the technocrats of the horrible future, then obviously any amount of money spent on this project would be well spent.

DENISE LEVERTOV   I've always believed that compassion is a function of the imagination, because without imagination how can you put yourself in the other fellow's boots? So anything which stimulates the imagination is capable of stimulating compassion, which would otherwise remain an undeveloped faculty.

I think it's a basic human potential. It can be developed. It can also be undeveloped. It can be in abeyance. It can be atrophied, like anything that is not used. I don't think it can be developed by reading literature alone, but I think that reading literature can be a contributing factor and a very important one.

NANCY ANDREASEN   One of the most important factors in developing compassion in medical students is to have good role models. Historically, the old doctors were better educated, read more literature than the new doctors, and were much more compassionate. But of course another variable intervenes here. Years ago doctors had very little to offer except compassion.

JIM COWAN   Aren't we also talking about empathy? Empathy (as opposed to "bleeding" every time one's patients bleed) ought to be something that doctors could learn. And isn't this related to the sort of "warm objectivity" Denise was discussing earlier?

BILL OBER   Compassion in medicine is based on doctors' judgments about how much their patients can take. Sometimes it's better to tell the tale all at once, to be blunt. Sometimes the truth needs to be parceled out over a period of time.

DENISE LEVERTOV   But that's not compassion at all. That's the operation of common sense. The compassion comes in before with the realization of the patient's feelings. What to do about it is the common sense part.

It is essential when thinking about how to teach compassion to consider reinforcement. Of course it's not literature alone or listening to Beethoven's *Quartets*, or role models, or any of these things alone. It's a combination of factors surely, each reinforcing the others.

ELIZABETH SEWELL   Compassion involves a certain consciousness about the self, too. It's a readiness to watch yourself and see what you're doing—I don't know whether literature enhances this condition—but people are so extraordinarily unobservant about themselves.

DENISE LEVERTOV I think literature does encourage this self-consciousness. Literature does precisely that.

JO TRAUTMANN You know, my experience of teaching literature to medical students has shown me that they are more receptive than English majors—certainly English graduate students—to reading literature in the ways Jim's comments have suggested. Medical students seem willing to make literature work for them. In fact, they are so inundated that they insist on it.

DICK SELZER In most respects medical students are not different from other students, as doctors are not different from other people. But there are two special factors in the development of a doctor. One is guilt. We doctors swim in a sea of guilt all day and all night. It is because we have to lay a hand on people, and we fear some complication may arise as a result of our actions. A surgeon is created on the wreckage of a legion of patients who have survived his mistakes. Whereas we hate our guilt, and it is painful for us to endure day after day, we need it. Because without that guilt we are liable, as a group, to run riot on the populace.

The other related factor is self-protection. By God, we have to protect ourselves! When we cut into our patients—Jim is right—our own flesh must not bleed! We must surround ourselves with callouses so that we cannot feel the sharp prick and sting of what we do. Consequently, the stereotyped surgeon with the tough exterior emerges. In every Western movie ever made, the alcoholic doctor is dragged out of the saloon to cut a bullet out of the sheriff's thigh. I sympathize with that surgeon who is drunk all the time. If it isn't from literature that we in medicine are going to be comforted and given the strength and energy to pursue this dreadful task, then where are we going to get it?

BILL OBER I think you're making physicians out to be frailer vessels than they are.

DICK SELZER I was speaking of physicians as I wish them to be.

ELIZABETH SEWELL I'm having a little trouble with your word "guilt." What you're reacting to is a calling to a profession of real power. Anybody who is realistic and who has power knows perfectly well that he does a great deal of damage and has done it very mysteriously. One does the worst things to people, very often, through the best one has. It's the gift of yourself that can destroy people, not the mistakes. Oh, they are there too. I know about the mistakes and the failures. But I think that we who are teachers and writers and therefore those who know about power might have something to say to you doctors and your situation, and the other way around. The guilt may be a response to power. But the answer is not to abdicate the power.

BILL OBER   I don't doubt that the guilt is real for you, Dick. But pathologists don't have the same feelings. A good batting average for a surgeon might be 350, maybe higher. A pathologist doesn't have a batting average and his fielding average, even if he's not a particularly intelligent pathologist, is about 960. "Guilt" to me is inappropriate, exaggerated, with just a little too much valence in it.

NANCY ANDREASEN   Oh, "guilt" is the appropriate word, all right.

BILL OBER   Maybe my lack of guilt explains my boredom. But that's a private problem.

THE TENTH DIALOGIST   Getting back to power, I think medicine is something of a special case in that most forms of power operate at at least one remove. President Ford has power. President Ford is not personally looking at the dead Marines or Cambodians. Some teachers have power, but they're not likely ever to know what effect it has. The physician is like the soldier of an earlier generation, who personally had to witness the power of his bayonet, as opposed to the bombardier. For this reason, what we are calling compassion (what I would rather call the ability to believe in the reality of other people) is to some extent built into medicine. It's what produces Dick's bad nights and Nancy's.

NANCY ANDREASEN   Another thing which produces the guilt is

that there are no clearly right answers in medicine. Often in psychiatry one is choosing between two evils.

JO TRAUTMANN   Yes, *Equus*⁵ illustrates that beautifully. But perhaps we have decided against talking about literature which merely illustrates medical issues?

DENISE LEVERTOV   Well, I would like Elizabeth to talk a little more about how teachers have power. If we're going to talk about the analogies between literature and medicine—and thus, the usefulness of literature to medicine—then we have to understand better the power that writers and teachers of literature have.

ELIZABETH SEWELL   I'm going to say quite frankly that most teachers don't have any power at all, and don't want it. I think of the power as essentially magical, and I don't mean that in any whimsical way. Like all powers, it can be good for students or it can be bad for them. One can seduce students into thinking that they, too, can operate in this magical world. It's rather like the sorcerer's apprentice in that they dissipate or develop illusions about their own real sources of power. One does not try to draw students towards oneself, to say "Be like me, come be my disciple."

Then there are cases in which the power doesn't emanate from the self but rather from the literary material. The teacher here is asking students to commit themselves to the power. For instance, I've seen the reading of a work of William Blake knock somebody clear out of his sanity. That's the kind of thing I mean. Teachers and writers can have magical power, which is rather different—though not wholly different—from doctors' power.

AL VASTYAN   What do you mean by "magical power"?

ELIZABETH SEWELL   It's a power I'm very aware of, and which I'm sure we all possess; however, I do not understand it very well and I would like to know much more about it. I'm beginning really to work with magic now.

DICK SELZER   Is it the same magic that takes place in the theatre?

ELIZABETH SEWELL   Yes, yes, it is. Exactly that magic. You can feel it rise and fall, and when it slacks, people cough and shuffle their feet. Music has it too, and it only works person-to-person. It doesn't work for me with movies or television. And I want to say that the lack of this sort of magic is a disaster for education because without it nothing happens except routine instruction. Coleridge says the aim of education is to elicit power in your students, to make them aware of their own powers. I love that. I think it's true and that it can be very dangerous.

AL VASTYAN   You know, words have been used here today that remind me of a remarkable essay by Carl Rogers in which he talks about the necessary and sufficient conditions of the helping relationship.[6] He says there are three and only three. The first is accurate empathy, and "accurate" is the key word.

ELIZABETH SEWELL   "Correct compassion."[7]

DENISE LEVERTOV   Yes, that's a beautiful poem.

AL VASTYAN   And the second element is congruence, in which if the so-called "helper" cannot manifest what he is feeling at the time, he must at least be aware of it. The third is nonpossessive warmth, or what Rogers calls love. I think these three are characteristic of a good teaching relationship, or a doctor-patient relationship; and I think this is what good literature does, too.

DENISE LEVERTOV   "Nonpossessive warmth"—that's probably what I meant by objectivity that is not cold.

24 May 1975

JO TRAUTMANN   You have all met Ian Lawson, who joined us last night, and breakfasted with us this morning, but you have not yet had a chance to hear the particular concerns he has brought to this dialogue. They are quite different from what we were talking about yesterday. Ian is interested in language and some of the philosophical problems in medicine today which have to do with language.

IAN LAWSON   To deal with the complexities of patient care in modern American society, one has to put together some fairly complicated resources, so that doctors can end up being institutional engineers. I have been in the States about five or six years, ostensibly working in the care of the elderly. I have become increasingly aware that it's not the biology of the elderly that's the problem, but the dysfunctional cybernetics or the arrangements that the able-bodied and able-minded create around the disabled.

A particular and very contemporary focus of that situation is what's happening to the language of medical care under two pressures: first, the pressure of having to extend language to cover the complicated biology of elderly and multiply disabled people; and second, the pressure of public accountability, such as PSRO [Professional Standards Review Organization].

The elderly represent the most extraordinary heterogeneity—unique profiles, unstable profiles, all in what seems at first to be an inextricable mishmash of social and environmental circumstances (for instance, the daughter-in-law in Chicago who has a sick baby) mixed with intervening support systems. This statement is somewhat explosive if one's only perception of medical language is what could be contained in the system known as the International Classification of Disease. Alvan Feinstein, in his various writings on the taxonomy of illness,[8] points out that what we use in language is frequently a derivative from the autopsy table and not in fact a language created around the *in vivo* realities of sick people. In his essay on nosography,[9] Francis Walshe noted that "in nature there are no diseases; there are only sick people."

There is a new and enormous pressure to use summary labels of diseases. At our institution we use instead a version of Lawrence Weed's Problem-Oriented Medical Record[10] to come closer to describing the complicated situations of our patients. But being this descriptive does not reduce tensions—it creates them. For when the Medicare authorities ask for the reason for a particular treatment, we send them copies of our records. This procedure is only the beginning of a ridiculous amount of paperwork, and I tell them, "I'm not here to educate the insurance system!" Furthermore, as a result of PSRO, we are going to have to say how much care a person gets based on a single item of information. We are setting up norms and criteria for "disease-related eligibility." Therefore, if you come to the health care system with a specific disease label, you will be told as a physician or a patient: "the median in this area for this condition is ten days; with certain complications, ten days plus two." In the use of medical language, the temptation has always been to reduce the amount of verbiage and this distresses me, for I am convinced that as you speak, so do you act.

I feel like a terrier who's down a rabbit hole. It's dark, but it's interesting. There are intriguing antagonisms down there, and I can't see what they are. Whether you can pull me out by the tail and say, "Look, there are some helpful parallels in literature," I really don't know.

ELIZABETH SEWELL   This is enormously interesting to me because taxonomy is one of the functions of poetry. And I found myself thinking of Eichmann as a sort of medical-legal problem. Eichmann apparently thought exclusively in clichés. Should we recognize the Eichmanns among us by their language? I'm thinking of language as a symptom here—hmm, you've opened up much too much!

GENE MOSS   There are two questions I'd like to raise. One, to what extent is this method of disposing of a patient population a self-conscious, studied method?

NANCY ANDREASEN   You don't mean "disposing"?

GENE MOSS   Yes, I mean disposing of a problem, getting it out of sight, out of mind.

BILL OBER   Off your desk.

GENE MOSS   Exactly. It's so much easier to write down one cryptic phrase with the clear knowledge that the cost-benefit ratio when dealing with someone at age seventy is far different from dealing with someone at age thirty. I wonder if this phenomenon isn't understood and accepted by, say, Blue Cross and Blue Shield and by others who deliver health care when dealing with someone whose benefit to society is minimal.

My second question concerns the larger issue of "naming"

in the patient-physician relationship. I've been impressed with E. Fuller Torrey's book[11] in which he discusses the dependence on a shared language that has mysterious qualities for the patient. This language is seen as an essential ingredient in an effective relationship between patient and doctor. It's an act of faith on the part of the patient in subscribing to a language that he only partly understands, but which comforts him. What is troubling him is not chaotic, but can be known, defined, handled by a word or a cluster of words which are specialist in nature, magical almost. I wonder how much pressure is involved here to reduce long descriptive analyses to a collection of special terms. Such long analyses seem far too much like the disorganized experience one feels when ill.

BILL OBER   The purpose of filling out a Blue Cross/Blue Shield form is to get a check. It needn't even be a very accurate description of the patient. It's neither an exercise in medicine nor literature, but merely a matter of bookkeeping.

JO TRAUTMANN   I think the time has come to consider explicitly what directions we want this dialogue to take.

GENE MOSS   To supply some sense of agenda: am I right in seeing a confluence of interest in "madness and art" as a guide for our discussion at the next meeting? We seem to have two or three people interested in addressing that subject.

DENISE LEVERTOV   Fine. And there should be a second theme suggested by the people who don't particularly want to talk about madness and art.

JIM COWAN   Another topic which interests *me* is one which Dick raised—I mean "the body." He writes about it from the standpoint of the surgeon. And I'd like to approach the topic from some of the ideas in D. H. Lawrence's work.

ELIZABETH SEWELL   It still seems to me that one of the necessary dimensions of our talk will have to be thinking about what *health* is.

JO TRAUTMANN   The definition of health is something which the philosophers and social scientists have been working on for years. What sorts of special contributions to the issue do you see literature making?

ELIZABETH SEWELL I don't know. I work by prophecy, not by prediction.

One of the tensions usually noticeable at the beginning of interdisciplinary dialogues was happily absent here. There was no inhibiting awe. The people from medicine did not feel that they were in the presence of the "keepers of beauty and truth"; nor did the literature teachers and writers feel they were in the presence of the "white knights of action." There was, to be sure, a bit of reverential bowing in each other's direction, but it was not of the sort to slow down the search for what everyone had in common.

The real ceremony was going on at another level. The dialogists kept up a regular rhythmic motion towards the point at which barriers could be surmounted. Several times the group collectively moved towards that amalgamation which could be recognized as a new idea, that illumination so bright as to be an epiphany, only to move just as steadily away again. Epiphanies are disturbing when one is alone, but they can be downright embarrassing in front of strangers. Furthermore, each dialogist, no doubt to varying degrees, thought it a matter of intellectual integrity to speak from within the boundaries of the discipline(s) he or she brought to the meeting. Even Elizabeth Sewell, who said early that literature was far too important and of too large a scope to be left exclusively to English departments, later imaged her relationship with Ian Lawson as two people, each stuck in a hole of his/her own, drumming loudly in an attempt to communicate with the other across the way.

One of the threatening aspects of that barrier towards which the group first moved and then retreated was the fear that beyond it might lie the land of the nebulous. The literary people in the group had a love for definite form and for controlling situations through the use of words. So when someone suggested that the primary act of both pathology and literary criticism was identifying patterns, he knocked a chink out of the barrier. When through this hole came streaming the probability that every-thing implied by the term "structuralism" might be helpful to the dialogue, and the possibility that Everything would be help-ful, we backed off again.

We would return only when we were ready. We had first to consider our duty at hand: what in literature would be valuable for a course at a college of medicine? Which pieces of literature illustrate medical concerns? [12] We had to discuss a topic, mad-ness and art, which we knew for certain had great importance in both literature and medicine. In other words, we would make more detailed maps of a territory we already knew a little of, and then we would proceed to a slightly stranger topic, the body. In the meantime, the tenth dialogist, calling himself a futurist, jumped over the barrier and was hurried on by who knows what fate.

Madness and Art
The Body
Literature vs. Medicine

17 October 1975

The subject of madness and art provoked from Nancy Andreasen a paper in which she made a strong plea for classical, as opposed to romantic, values in life, if not necessarily in literature. She reminded the other dialogists that "confessional" writers like Robert Lowell, Sylvia Plath, and Anne Sexton had experienced serious mental illness and that the last two had killed themselves. She asserted that we ought in no sense to romanticize mental illness as a predictable and even essential corollary of genius.

Thinking about Anne Sexton's death, Denise Levertov had recently written an essay which addressed our subject of madness and art in ways complementary to Nancy's. That essay was circulated among the group.[1]

There were a few murmurings against the stand taken by Nancy and Denise. No one advanced the outrageously sentimental notion that madness in artists ought to be left untreated. But Jim Cowan, for one, suspected that Nancy's psychiatric practice was too rigidly scientific for him. Jim believed she did not have faith in what he considered to be the self-evident value of dynamic therapy. Jo Trautmann, for another, in a pre-meeting letter to the group, had cited the instance of Virginia Woolf as one in whom the relationship between madness and art was perhaps

creative. Jo had not wanted to play down the pain of mental illness or to ignore the very real problem of self-destructiveness in
artists, but rather intended to suggest that the situation was not
as easy as Nancy and Denise apparently assumed.

In another letter, Elizabeth Sewell rejected the entire subject
of madness and art as central to our dialogue: "I do not draw the
line between medicine and literature—a line of interaction and
polarity and delight—at any point where studies of writers' sex-
lives, neuroses, psychoses, suicidal acts or tendencies, writers'
medical histories are anything other than peripheral."

Gene Moss liked the tenor of Nancy's thoughts on the subject,
but was inclined to broaden the topic of madness in artists to
include several other categories not often considered. Spurred on
by the talk at Meeting Two, Gene produced a paper for Meeting
Four in which he discussed these expansions.

Bill Ober contributed an impressive scholarly investigation
into the concept of "spleen," the organ traditionally associated
with melancholy, and simultaneously demonstrated how the
historical method can bring literature and medicine together.[2]
Amidst all these exchanges, formal and informal, Nancy's was
central.

SUFFERING AND ART: A DEFENSE OF SANITY,
by Nancy C. Andreasen

. . . men must learn by suffering.
Drop by drop in sleep upon the heart
Falls the laborious memory of pain,
Against one's will comes wisdom.
The grace of the gods is forced on us,
Throned inviolably.

Aeschylus, *Agamemnon*

Those lines from Aeschylus still have the same fresh-
ness and power for the twentieth century that they had when he
wrote them some 2500 years ago. The problem of suffering—its
meaning or purpose in a blankly unjust and sometimes malig-
nant world—has been a concern for centuries. The nature of the
problem rests on the assumption that suffering per se is an evil

which must somehow be justified. To make suffering endurable, since it is also capriciously inevitable, people have tried to find reasons why it might contain a kernel or two of goodness as well. Though the means are evil, the end might be a good. Aeschylus's reason, the concept of *pathei mathos*, is one of the more cogent: suffering has an awful value in that through it men may learn, grow, or become strengthened. But despite the power of Aeschylus' poetry and the cogency of his reasoning, most people would prefer to remain small and stupid and weak rather than endure terrible suffering. Reasons are sought only for purposes of consolation. Few actually seek suffering in order to become strong or noble.

A person or an era in which those priorities become turned around is in trouble. Such an erroneous reordering of priorities is at present plaguing modern writing with perverse results. Suffering has been romantically and pathologically glorified as an end in itself. Too many aspiring or even successful writers seem to believe that to be creative one should perhaps seek out suffering, that to be a writer one must inevitably suffer. "The suffering poet" has become an ideal model. And suicide has even become glorified as a fitting self-immolation to the Muses. But instead the Muses may find the sacrificial fumes rather unsavory. Martyrdom should be the accidental consequence of pursuing a high goal rather than a good to be sought after for itself. Suffering well may make a person a saint, but never an artist.

Historical Roots: Recent

The modern group of writers who have publicized the association between suffering and creativity or madness and creativity have been dubbed the "confessional school." The group is actually rather heterogeneous, including such figures as Sexton, Lowell, and Plath. Its members primarily share the bond that they have suffered from psychiatric illness (predominantly depression), have been hospitalized for the illness, and have chosen to use their personal emotional experiences as subject matter for their poetry.

Robert Lowell is in a sense the founding father of the school, his *Life Studies* setting the precedent in 1959 with a grim account of his experiences while hospitalized for depression at McLean. In "Waking in the Blue," he describes the early morning sleep disturbance which frequently occurs in depression.

The night attendant, a B.U.
sophomore, rouses from the mare's
nest of his drowsy head propped on
The Meaning of Meaning.
He catwalks down our corridor.
Azure day
makes my agonized blue window bleaker.
Crows maunder on the petrified fairway.
Absence! My heart grows tense
as though a harpoon were sparring
for the kill.
(This is the house for the
"mentally ill.")

The confessions of Lowell tend to be tightly written, with the wry irony of a New England blueblood too proud to submerge himself in pathos. One might argue that his return to highly personal subject matter, and in particular his advocacy of feelings and emotions as fit subject matter for poetry, provided a necessary and inevitable liberation from the harsh dry intellectualism of the Eliot era. That argument, often presented, tends to be over-simplistic: Robert Frost and W. H. Auden often used emotional responses as both nidus and subject for poems during the Eliot era. But T. S. Eliot, not Frost and Auden, was the poet most likely to be imitated and admired by younger writers.

Lowell's precedent *was* imitated. For a time Boston University became the center of a coterie. Lowell's position had obviously struck sympathetic chords in other writers and readers. Literary heroes only a few years earlier had typically been mystical (like William Butler Yeats), or iconoclastic (like James Joyce), or entrenched in tradition (like Eliot). Dylan Thomas, a hero in his drunken self-destructiveness, was a forewarning of this new era. But in the sixties the trend became a movement. To be a writer it seemed that one must be a suffering writer, painfully lost in a dark wood of despair and self-destruction. Experimenting with drugs and suicide provided a kind of entry into the new literary club. Seeking or requiring psychiatric treatment was another admission ticket.

This glorification of suffering or madness reflects the exaggeration of an attitude common among intellectuals and literati for many years. Particularly on the East coast, to be "in analysis" has been a badge of sensitivity. Its snob appeal has been based on the facts that psychoanalysts usually accept intelligent and articulate patients who are wealthy enough to afford a minimum of three hours of treatment per week and healthy enough to endure intensive self-exploration. Thus patients in analysis are usually drawn from the intellectual and social elite. Only a small extension of traditional attitudes was required to certify as elite those who had been treated as inpatients as well as those who had been treated as outpatients. If the persons being analyzed are sensitive and brave, then those who have been hospitalized for their conditions must have even greater sensitivity and greater insights. But just as Eliot must have objected to his followers who "got religion" for the wrong reasons, so Lowell and Plath and Sexton would probably have objected to their admirers who "got depressed."

Perhaps it is time to present another point of view about the value and significance of psychiatric treatment, one which some of the "confessional poets" might even share. In contrast to European psychiatry, American psychiatry has been based primarily on Freudian psychodynamic theory for many years. Psychodynamic theory tends to follow a "psychological model" to describe the causes and treatments for emotional problems. Its premise, which has had enormous appeal, is that people could achieve greater health and strength if they break down their personalities under the intensive self-examination of psychoanalysis, recognize sick or neurotic aspects, and then rebuild their personalities, now free from neurotic traits. Problems so distant as starvation, political dissension, pollution, or inflation are too serious to be solved by individuals. But psychodynamic theory offers a chance to solve one's own problems at least.

This point of view, which has dominated psychiatry in the United States until recent years, has coexisted with another theory predominant in Europe. Although Austria and Switzerland, as homelands for psychodynamic theory, have tended to follow it, Germany, England, and France have chosen instead to follow the competing "medical model." The medical model asserts that psychiatry treats *illnesses*, just as other medical specialties do, and that its achievements must necessarily be rather modest. This model suggests that medicine can offer a stay of execution, a hope that life can be prolonged with some attendant suffering, but it can seldom promise total health and well-being. The model also applies to psychiatric illnesses such as schizophrenia, obsessive-compulsive disorder, or depression. Based on the work of men like Freud's respected German contemporary, Emil Kraepelin, the medical model in psychiatry stresses that illnesses of psychiatric patients can be treated, and their symptoms often improved, but that cures should rarely be promised.

The medical model puts things in a useful perspective. Psychiatric illnesses, presumed ultimately to be diseases of the brain occurring at the biochemical level, are not diseases of the psyche or soul. One cannot romanticize or sentimentalize about them any more than one can about diabetes or cancer. Talking with psychiatric patients might help them feel better. (It will usually help patients with cancer feel better, too.) Medication may remove many irritating symptoms such as the insomnia of depression or the auditory hallucinations of schizophrenia, but taking medication is not usually pleasant and certainly not a panacea. Sometimes the illness remits for long periods and sometimes blessedly for the remainder of the patient's life. When that situation occurs, both doctor and patient feel grateful indeed.

The psychodynamic point of view epitomized by Freud seems in some ways closer to religion than medicine: its goal is self-improvement and self-fulfillment; redemption is promised in the form of complete mental health to those who seek treatment. The medical model offers only diagnosis and treatment: the doctor extends a hand to the patient and offers whatever help is possible, knowing full well that it may not be enough to make either of them happy.

Historical Roots: Distant

Thus in some respects the tendency to romanticize and glorify psychiatric illness and treatment has been a recent development. Although many Freudians would vehemently disavow this romanticization, the popularity of psychodynamic theories in America has had a significant influence on recent developments in American literature. Perhaps, in fact, the widespread acceptance of Freudian theory in America but not in Europe may partially explain why the glorification of the suffering writer has been primarily an American movement and the many recent suicides of literary personages have all been American.

But of course nothing is quite so patently simple. Questions about the value of suffering have been with us as long as suffering itself. To determine how and why glorification of suffering became a problem, it might be helpful to sample some of the various answers given to such questions.

Perhaps because the struggle to survive was so painfully real, there was no problem with the glorification of suffering in the classical period. Various writers—classical tragedians and biblical authors alike—ask why humanity must suffer, and particularly why people must suffer when innocent, when in pursuit of justice, or when seeking purity. Tragic protagonists—Job, Antigone, Agamemnon, Hippolytus—reflect various confrontations with the question. The answers are diverse: God or the gods test man's mettle with suffering; the proud to some extent bring suffering upon themselves; suffering heroes grow wiser and more human through experiencing pain. The classical period thus imparted *pathei mathos* as an attitude about suffering. Suffering, an awful burden, must be borne courageously because learning and growth come through experiencing it.

Although generalizations can be made about suffering heroes, suffering writers of the classical period remain somewhat of an enigma. Aristotle remarked: "Those who have become eminent in philosophy, politics, poetry, and the arts have all had tendencies toward melancholia." Socrates, who did not write, is the only figure whose life has been recorded to any degree. He did suffer, was a martyr, and was admired for his martyrdom. It was his biographer Plato who sowed the first seeds for an escapist attitude which seeks refuge from the dark cave of pain and unreality that is life. But even so, Plato and Aristotle did not found a movement which implied that men should be admired because they suffered.

The Christian era, which followed chronologically and intellectually, did glorify suffering excessively in its early stages. For centuries, Christianity has balanced precariously between extremes of masochism and sublimation; the denial of life and the celebration of life; the world as a place of evil to be transcended and the world of God's creation and a reflection of His eminence; the body as a corrupt and decaying shell for the soul and the body as a lovely garment which the soul will don again at the resurrection. As portrayed in the New Testament, Jesus is himself ambiguous, seeing both sides of almost every issue possible, whether political, aesthetic, ethical, or metaphysical. That Christian tradition continues to espouse such a delicate equilibrium is no surprise and undoubtedly is one reason for Christianity's wide appeal.

However, early Christians were not so balanced. To them, life was evil, suffering sought after because our Lord suffered, and martyrdom valued. But as the Day of Judgment became a more and more distant possibility, the church fathers redefined things and made the glorification of suffering *as an end in itself* a heresy—whether the Donatist heresy of seeking martyrdom or the Manichaean heresy of seeing the world and the body as innately evil.

Although extremes had been moderated, attitudes toward suffering emerged with an emphasis different from those expressed in classical times. Medieval writings were distinctly pessimistic and otherworldly. Suffering and self-denial seemed appealing both because as in classical times, they served to strengthen individuals, and because they represented an imitation of Christ. Thus suffering was to some extent glorified—because it led to sainthood, not because it led to poetry.

In Renaissance literature a premonition of what would provide the basis for modern attitudes appeared. During the Jacobean period (late Renaissance), when the golden promises of the brave new world began to tarnish, an age of pessimism and melancholy evolved which is still apparent today. Archetypal notes are Shakespeare's depressive soliloquies in *Hamlet*; and Donne's *Death's Duell* delivered in the pulpit of St. Paul's and his posing in a shroud at home. While the classical period had viewed suffering as appalling and the medieval as a ladder to saintliness, the Renaissance judged it to be appealing as well as appalling.

Hamlet's internal debate about suicide is truly a touchstone. He wonders:

Whether 'tis nobler in the mind to suffer
The slings and arrows of outrageous fortune
Or to take arms against a sea of troubles,
And by opposing end them. To die, to sleep—
No more, and by a sleep to say we end
The heart-ache, and the thousand natural shocks
That flesh is heir to; 'tis a consummation
Devoutly to be wish'd.

(III.i.56—63)

Hamlet asks whether it is nobler to endure the terrible suffering of the depression which he is experiencing or to commit suicide. For the first time in many years both suicide and the experience of melancholy are ennobling.

However, both the character Hamlet and the play as a whole reach different conclusions about this issue than do the "confessional" writers of today. Suicide is ruled out as an unacceptable alternative almost immediately in the soliloquy. Hamlet becomes a redeemed and successful person only after his return from England when, having recovered from his melancholy, he can assume his responsibilities as his father's son and a prince of Denmark.

By and large this issue receded in the literature of the neoclassical period, erupting with new force during the Romantic period. It has been a force to be reckoned with ever since. A group of writers emerged who considered the purpose of life to be the expansion or enrichment of their individual human experience: art as the incarnation of such experience recollected in tranquility. The Romantic period provided artists with particularly colorful and interesting lives. But in spite of their disrupted, disruptive lives, their sometimes perverse and melancholic delight in appearing as the "suffering artist" or "doomed poet," the Romantic writers seldom were actively self-destructive. They died young, lamenting the fact of death, by disease and accident rather than by suicide. Nevertheless, it is only a small step from their stance to that of the "confessional poets." Both the Romantics and the "confessionals" share an emphasis on the pursuit of personal experience for its own sake, whatever the consequences, and the belief that personal experience is a rich and powerful resource for the creation of poetry.

Palpable Roots: Psychiatric

So strong an association as that between suffering and art obviously is based on reasons other than historic ones. That the relationship between genius and insanity has been discussed for centuries and occasionally taken as fact indicates that it must have some roots in reality. Psychiatric data examining the association varies enormously in quality and therefore in value. Much of the data deals with the more general subject of association between genius and mental illness rather than the specific subject of literary creativity and mental illness. Among the earliest modern writers on the subject was Cesare Lombroso, who in 1864 published *Genius and Insanity*,[3] in which he argued for the close association between those two entities. A variety of anecdotal volumes chronicling the decadent or crazed lives of various men of genius and their families followed Lombroso's precedent.[4] Any scientist is painfully aware of the deceptive ease with which anecdotal accounts can pass for proof and how difficult real proof is to achieve.

Subsequent investigators have attempted to examine the association between genius and insanity using quantitative methods. The "geniuses" studied have varied from Havelock Ellis's more broadly-defined group (including statesmen as well as poets) to Adele Juda's more specific definitions of various types of creativity, which focus particularly on artists.[5] Most of these investigations suggest that gifted individuals possibly have more psychiatric illness than other people. The fact that their relatives also tend to have more illness implies that creativity and psychiatric disorder could run together in families. However, none of these investigations examined writers as a specific group.

In my own study of writers at the University of Iowa Writers' Workshop, I tried to examine the prevalence of psychiatric symptoms in a group of poets and novelists.[6] This study documented specifically what its predecessors had already suggested. The writers interviewed had a much higher incidence of illness and treatment than did a matched control group: nine out of fifteen had seen a psychiatrist, eight had been treated, and four had been hospitalized. Most of them described symptoms which led to a diagnosis of mood disorder; two had both mania and depression, while eight had depression only. Six of them had symptoms of alcoholism, five of whom were also depressed. Their relatives also had a higher incidence of psychiatric symptoms and creativity than those of the control group. Twenty-one percent of the writers' relatives were given a psychiatric diagnosis, usually depression, in contrast to only 4 percent of the controls' relatives. Twenty-three percent were considered creatively gifted, in comparison to only 7 percent among the control group.

Although this study is far from definitive for a variety of reasons, it does corroborate experience and common sense at least in terms of the diagnosis given. Problems with depression and dependence on alcohol or drugs usually have troubled writers in the past: Donne, Virginia Woolf, Johnson, De Quincey, Coleridge, Keats come quickly to mind. Because psychiatric illness has become so fashionable, the rate of illness possibly is unusually high and may not reflect actual illness among writers through the centuries. On the other hand, a survey of past writers would inevitably lead to an underestimation because so much information has been lost through the passage of time.

In any case, if one were to choose the psychiatric illness most likely to be associated with creativity simply on the basis of common sense, it would probably be mood disorder. Schizophrenia, which has sometimes been considered a candidate in the past, tends to be too crippling, chronic, and incapacitating. But the person with mood disorder typically has peaks and valleys with prolonged normal periods in between, and except when the illness is very severe, he need not be totally incapacitated. In addition to never permanently impairing productivity and creativity because of its remitting course, mood disorder could conceivably even enhance creativity. Many individuals with mood disorder seem either unusually energetic or unusually sensitive between episodes, and either of these traits is an asset to the creative person. Furthermore, the experience of an illness such as depression or mania conceivably could increase a writer's insight into human experience and thereby enrich his creative resources.

Palpable Roots: The Challenges of Writing

Finding that writers suffer symptoms of depression more frequently than others does not reveal anything about cause and effect, although the familial pattern of inheritance could imply that mood disturbance is genetically determined and not caused by the challenges of writing. But in looking at the issue of the relationship between creativity and illness in reverse, it is possible to suggest that there is something about the nature of the creative act, particularly writing, which is intrinsically disturbing or painful and which may predispose to the development of depressive symptoms.

Many of the observations made here are based on interviews with workshop writers about the tensions they experienced as writers. Most described a nagging personal self-doubt and a delight in mastering these doubts, an interaction which could prod the creative process. Each time a writer approaches a blank sheet of paper, he places his artistic integrity on trial. Asked when he first began to believe he was a writer, one poet replied: "I'm still not sure. The standard by which I judge myself keeps going up." Such intensive self-criticism is not conducive to personal comfort or peace of mind, although it is likely to increase the quality of the art produced. Paradoxically, public recognition is important and yet never satisfying. When asked why he wrote, one writer commented "It's a drive for recognition, admiration, affection. It is the first way I was distinguished as a kid." But another indicated why the drive for recognition is also self-defeating: "If you're in competition with anyone, it's with yourself." Although each writer aspires "to be the best," his own internal critical arbiter—ultimately far harsher than the literary critics—insists the competition with aesthetic perfection (which can never be won because the standards keep going up) is more meaningful than competition with his peers.

All artists are on trial with each performance. In some ways the challenge and potential threats are greater in other media than in writing. If Michelangelo accidentally had broken off the hand of the Pieta as he was completing the masterpiece, two years of effort irreparably would have been lost. A Heifetz or a Sutherland must be up for each performance on a regular basis; there is no way of retracting a note once played or sung. The writer can at least work and rework until satisfied that he has achieved at a level acceptable to his standards. For a poet, if not for a novelist, the commitment can be brief, and only a little time and paper is lost if he rejects the final product for aesthetic reasons.

But writing differs from other art forms in ways that make it perhaps the most challenging and frightening of all. Although writing is the most human, personal, and interpersonal of all art forms, it is also incredibly lonely. In a very literal sense, the writer puts his life on the line. Asked how often they draw on personal experience for their subject matter, almost all of the writers admitted to doing so most of the time. (Some indicated that they could not imagine drawing on anything else, and others added that personal experience must be defined broadly, to include observation of and interaction with other people.) A majority also indicated that their work tended to grow out of personal conflict—although usually with the qualification that it be "conflict recollected in tranquility" if the appropriate emotional distance necessary to create art rather than maudlin sentimentality is to be reached. The writer must deal with himself and his experiences as both analyst and analysand. He must live them intensely, and yet also stand back, observe them critically, analyze rationally, and often judge harshly. The pain involved in self-analysis is well known to most psychiatrists. The writer's craft demands that he experience this pain and go on to make it public by transforming it into a work of art. As one of the writers commented, "My workshop students leave themselves incredibly open. Although they sometimes pretend that their works have nothing to do with their personal lives, you can see their problems and their pain transparently laid out in what they write."

Anyone who thinks writing simply involves self-revelation obviously is naïve. Nevertheless, writers must leave themselves more open than other artists because of the nature of the art form. Writing has a stark simplicity about it. Unlike the sculptor or the violinist, the writer's only instrument is himself. As he writes, he uses his mind and imagination to transform his own experience into words on paper which somehow will recreate for a future reader the complexity and pain of the human dilemma or the irony and joy of the human comedy. In the process of writing he must achieve a heightened state of sensitivity during which he relives imaginatively the emotions or experience he is re-creating. Thus his medium inevitably and continuously draws him closer to life, and to the tragedy or cruelty of life, than someone who is able to interpose a marble figure or a wordless sonata between himself and his audience.

In addition to producing continual inner tension, demanding a painful closeness to emotional life, and requiring that these burdens be carried in loneliness and isolation, writing provides in return few rewards. Public recognition is fickle and fortuitous. Working with timely topics or including liberal amounts of sexual material is more likely to produce a best seller, but good writers are usually not willing to sell out to a commercial goal. Unfortunately, however, they must either make enough through their writing to become independent financially or write part time while holding another job.

For the poet financial rewards are even fewer than for the novelist. Rarely can a poet become independent financially through the sale of his works. Thus most writers must experience a frustrating drain on creative energies when forced to take teaching jobs, give lectures, write journalistic pieces, or work in Hollywood. Although intermittently diverting and enjoyable at times, such activities interfere with the ultimate goal of most good writers: to create something genuinely fine, perhaps something that will be viable after their death.

A Defense of Sanity

Ours is still mostly a Romantic era, and classical values simply are not "in." Both the Romantic and the classical eras produced great artists. But which era produced better lives? That question is all the more relevant now, since readers and critics have become less willing to separate a writer's life from his art, and particularly in view of the toll of suicides the Romantic set has taken in recent years.

Speaking as a literary critic, I cannot answer the question of whether the value of art produced by the Romantic set of the "confessional school" outweighs the cost in lives and suffering. Their closeness chronologically makes it difficult to evaluate their work objectively. It is too early to know whether the widespread appeal of their work is a passing fad or whether its popularity will continue in another century.

Speaking as a psychiatrist and as a human being, I can offer an opinion on the significant dangers of idealizing psychiatric illness and suicide. I can make an appeal for a return to more classical attitudes toward both life and art for medical and psychological reasons, if not for aesthetic reasons. Taking the medical reasons first, to idealize mental illness and the powers of psychological analysis is simply unrealistic. Interest in psychology and psychiatry among lay people and among artists has grown out of proportion. People read opinion masquerading as fact and are often encouraged to diagnose and recommend treatment for themselves and others. Psychiatrists must take part of the blame for overestimating what they know and overselling what they can do. A nirvana of growth, understanding, and insight has been offered to patients. Such promises rarely can be kept. Some psychologists and psychiatrists have even joined in the romanticization and idealization of suffering and illness.

It is high time that someone made a more human claim for what the healing arts can offer. Psychiatric illnesses, like other illnesses, range from mild (warts and dandruff) to severe (cancer). Patients often can be very interesting people, but their illnesses are either a nuisance or, still worse, quite painful, noteworthy only to the extent that they are "interesting cases" of this or that condition. Real patients rarely find their depressions or their alcoholism fascinating. Just as real illness is far from appealing, so the level of treatment remains rather primitive and unpleasant. In spite of numerous prophetic and dogmatic pronouncements found in popular journals and at the paperback stands, almost nothing actually is known about the causes of mental illness, very little about definitive treatment, and barely anything about how to define it. Far from being able to offer a nirvana of growth and insight, psychiatrists do not even know much about how to improve the ordinary human lot of schizophrenia or personality disturbance.

Most real mental illness is painful or unappealing, hardly appropriate for romantic idealization and certainly not worth pursuing as a personal goal because it might increase insights or create an artist. In addition to being unsound for medical reasons (in that mental illness is unpleasant or drab rather than enriching or interesting), the romanticization of suffering and suicide is wrong on psychological grounds as well. The Romantic set in general places an emphasis on the value of personal experience at whatever the cost. "Self-realization" and "self-actualization" are the modern fashionable terms. (The old-fashioned word is probably "selfishness," an ugly, scolding word our parents used to use and which many of us would prefer to forget.) The risks of making self-enrichment the goal of life are enormous. At best this attitude leads to purposeless pleasure-seeking, imparting only impermanent relationships that often lead to the exploitation of other people. At worst the pursuit of self-realization expands experience in the form of masochistic self-destructiveness—often in the form of experimentation with drugs, suicidal behavior, or a self-pitying withdrawal into Weltschmerz.

Perhaps some people need to burst free from inhibitions, to learn to become more introspective, or to permit themselves more pleasure. But that is no longer a common problem in American society in the 1970s. Rather, too much emphasis on understanding or actualizing the self is the problem. People come to the psychiatrist wanting to "find themselves." Self-realization is not achieved by looking at the abyss of painful past experiences or present suffering, but by looking out at others and using past experiences as a reservoir to understand or comfort them. Self-affirmation is not achieved by suffering and suicide. The Romantic set which has glorified self-discovery generally and the experience of suffering in particular is dangerous and destructive—and wrong.

Creative writers are torchbearers of civilization. In recent years many have been unable to complete their marathon. Powerful writers have led compelling lives, struggled with mental illness, but finally given in to its pain and destroyed themselves through drugs or alcohol or suicide. Such powerful people set powerful examples. It is easy to assume that their suffering was a necessary and sufficient cause for their art. It was not. Suffering can be enriching, but never when pursued as an end in itself, and it can often be destructive. The torch they carried was their art, not their lives. It will advance civilization only to the extent that it sheds the light of sanity rather than insanity.

17 October 1975, Evening Session

After a day-long discussion of Nancy's paper together with the other essays on madness and art, the dialogists went to dinner, amused to find on the table several bottles of a wine called Chateau du Spleen, presented by Bill Ober as an augmentation to his paper. The wine was cheerfully consumed but had its splenetic effects on the after-dinner session.

JO TRAUTMANN   To begin our discussion of the body in literature and medicine, I have asked Dick Selzer to read us some of his work.

DICK SELZER *(reading)*   In the foyer of a great medical school, there hangs a painting of Vesalius.[7] Lean, ascetic, possessed, the anatomist stands before a dissecting table upon which lies the naked body of a man. The flesh of the two is silvery. A concentration of moonlight, like a strange rain of virus, washes them. The cadaver has dignity and reserve; it is distanced by its death. Vesalius reaches for his dissecting knife. As he does so, he glances over his shoulder at a crucifix on the wall. His face wears an expression of guilt and melancholy and fear. He knows that there is something wrong, forbidden in what he is about to do, but he cannot help himself, for he is a fanatic. He is driven by a dark desire. To see, to feel, to discover is all. His is a passion, not a romance.

I understand you, Vesalius. Even now, after so many voyages within, so much exploration, I feel the same sense, that one must not gaze into the body, the same irrational fear that it is an evil deed for which punishment awaits. Consider. The sight of our internal organs is denied us. To how many men is it given to look upon their own spleens, their hearts, and still live? The hidden geography of the body is a Medusa's head one glimpse of which would render blind the presumptuous eye. Still, rigid rules are broken by the smallest inadvertencies: I pause in the midst of an operation being performed under spinal anesthesia to observe the face of my patient, to speak a word or two of reassurance. I peer above the screen which separates his head from the abdomen in which I am most deeply employed. He is not asleep, but rather stares straight upward, his attention riveted, a look of terrible discovery, of wonder upon his face. Watch him. This man is violating a taboo. I follow his gaze upward, and see in the great operating lamp suspended above his belly the reflection of his viscera. There is the liver, dark and turgid above, there the loops of his bowel winding slow, there his blood runs expensively. It is that which he sees and studies with so much horror and fascination. Something primordial in him has been aroused—a fright, a longing. I feel it too, and quickly bend above his open body to shield it from his view. How dare he look within the Ark! Cover his eyes! But it is too late; he has already *seen*; that which no man should; he has trespassed. And I am no longer a surgeon, but a hierophant who must do magic to ward off the punishment of the angry Gods.

I feel some hesitation to invite you to come with me into the body. It seems a reckless, defiant act. Yet there is more than dread reflected from these rosy coasts, these restless estuaries of pearl. And it is time to share it, the way the catbird shares the song which must be a joy to him, and is a living truth to those who hear it. So shall I make of my fingers, words; of my scalpel, a sentence; of the body of my patient, a story.

One enters the body in surgery, as in love, as though one were an exile returning at last to his hearth, daring uncharted darkness in order to reach home. Turn sideways, if you will, and slip with me into the cleft I have made. Do not fear the yellow meadows of fat, the red that sweats and trickles where you step. Here, give me your hand. Lower between the beefy cliffs. Now rest a bit upon the peritoneum. All at once, gleaming, the membrane parts—and you are *in*.

It is the stillest place that ever was. As though suddenly you are struck deaf. Why, when the blood sluices fierce as Niagara, when the brain teems with electricity, and the numberless cells exchange their goods in ceaseless commerce—why is it so quiet? Has some priest in charge of these rites uttered the command "Silence"? This is no silence of the vacant stratosphere, but the awful quiet of ruins, of rainbows, full of expectation and holy dread. Soon you shall know surgery as a Mass served with Body and Blood, wherein disease is assailed as though it were sin.

Touch the great artery. Feel it bound like a deer in the might of its lightness, and know the thunderless boil of the blood. Lean for a bit against this bone. It is the only memento you will leave to the earth. Its tacitness is everlasting. In the hush of the tissue wait with me for the shaft of pronouncement. Press your ear against this body, the way you did as a child holding a seashell and heard faintly the half-remembered, longed-for sea. Now strain to listen *past* the silence. In the canals, cilia paddle quiet as an Iroquois canoe. Somewhere nearby a white whipslide of tendon bows across a joint. Fire burns here but does not crackle. Again, listen. Now there *is* sound—small splashings, tunnelled currents of air; slow gaseous bubbles ascend through dark, unlit lakes. Across the diaphragm and into the chest—here at last it is all noise; the whisper of the lungs, the *lubdup*, *lubdup* of the garrulous heart.

But it is good you do not hear the machinery of your marrow lest it madden like the buzzing of a thousand coppery bees. It is frightening to lie with your ear in the pillow, and hear the beating of your heart. Not that it beats—but that it might stop, even as you listen. For anything that moves must come to rest; no rhythm is endless but must one day lurch—then halt. Not that it is a disservice to a man to be made mindful of his death, but—at three o'clock in the morning it is less than philosophy. It is Fantasy, replete with dreadful images forming in the smoke of alabaster crematoria. It is then that one thinks of the bristle-cone pines, and envies them for having lasted. It is their slowness, I think. Slow down, heart, and drub on.

What is to one man a coincidence is to another a miracle. It was one or the other of these that I saw last spring. While the rest of Nature had agreed to the dismantling of Winter, Joe Riker remained obstinate through the change of the seasons. "No operation," said Joe, "I don't want no operation."

Joe Riker is a short-order cook in a diner where I sometimes drink coffee. Each week for six months he had paid a visit to my office, carrying his affliction like a pet mouse under his hat. Every Thursday at four o'clock he would sit on my examining table, lift the fedora from his head, and bend forward to show me the hole. He had a formal delicate way of taking off that hat—holding the brim on either side with thumbs and forefingers, whilst the fifth fingers of his hands were little wings extended. So that the hat seemed to take flight, be borne aloft, then slowly to settle like a gray pigeon upon his knees. Joe Riker's hole was as big as his mouth. You could have dropped a plum in it. Gouged from the tonsured top of his head, was a mucky puddle whose meaty heaped edge rose above the normal scalp about it. There was no mistaking the announcement from this rampart.

The cancer had chewed through Joe's scalp, munched his skull, then opened the membranes underneath—the dura mater, the pia mater, the arachnoid—until it had laid bare this short-order cook's brain, pink and gray, and pulsating, so with each beat a little pool of cerebral fluid quivered. Now and then a drop would manage the rim to run across his balding head, and Joe would reach one burry hand up to wipe away a tear. Each time I would see it, I must stifle anew my awe.

I would gaze then upon Joe Riker and marvel. How dignified he was, as though that tumor, gnawing him, denuding his very brain, had given him a grace that a lifetime of good health had not lent.

"Joe," I say, "let's get rid of it. Cut out the bad part, put in a metal plate, and you're cured." And I wait.

"No operation," says Joe. I try again.

"What do you mean 'no operation'? You're going to get meningitis. Any day now. And die. That thing is going to get to your brain." I think of it devouring the man's dreams and memories. I wonder what they are. The surgeon knows all the parts of the brain, but he does not know his patient's dreams and memories. And for a moment I am tempted—to take the man's head in my hands, hold it to my ear, and listen as I would to a seashell. But his dreams are none of my business. It is his flesh that matters.

"No operation," says Joe.

"You give me a headache," I say. And we smile, not because

the joke is funny anymore, but because we've got something between us, like a secret.

"Same time next week?" Joe asks. I wash out the wound with peroxide, and apply a dressing. He lowers the fedora over it.

"Yes," I say, "same time." And the next week he comes again.

There came the week when Joe Riker did not show up; nor did he the week after that, nor for a whole month. I drive over to his diner. He is behind the counter, shuffling back and forth between the grille and the sink. He is wearing the fedora. He sets a cup of coffee in front of me.

"I want to see your hole," I say.

"Which one?" he says, and winks.

"Never mind that," I say, "I want to see it." I am all business.

"Not here," says Joe. He looks around, checking the counter as though I have made an indecent suggestion.

"My office at four o'clock," I say.

"Yeah," says Joe, and turns away.

He is late. Everyone else has gone for the day. Joe is beginning to make me angry. At last he arrives.

"Take off your hat," I say, and he knows by my voice that I am not happy. He does, though, raises it straight up with both hands the way he always does, and I see—that the wound is healed. Where once there had been a bitten-out excavation, moist and shaggy, there is now a fragile bridge of shiny new skin. It has healed!

"What happened?" I manage.

"You mean that?" He points to the top of his head. "Oh well," he says, "the wife's sister, she went to France, and brought me a bottle of water from Lourdes. I've been washing it out with that for a month."

"Holy water?" I say.

"Yeah," says Joe. "Holy water."

At precisely that moment the sun breaks through the clouds and strikes the wall over my examining table. All the colors of the rainbow dance on that wall, and the room is bathed in its radiance.

Joe Riker? I see him now and then at the diner. He looks like anything but a fleshly garden of miracles. Rather he has taken on a terrible ordinariness—Eden after the Fall, and minus its most beautiful creatures. There is a certain bodily sloven, a dishevelment of the tissues. Perhaps I am wrong. Perhaps it is just the sly wink with which he greets me, as though to signal that we have shared something furtive, like sex. Or *was* it the disease which had ennobled him, and now that it was gone, he was somehow diminished by too much? Could such a man, I think as I sip my coffee, could such a man have felt the brush of wings? How often it seems that the glory leaves as soon as the wound is healed. But then it is only saints who bloom in martyrdom, becoming less and less the flesh that pains, more and more ghost-colored weightlessness.

It was many years between my first sight of the living human brain, and Joe Riker's windowing. I had thought then, long ago: Could this one-pound loaf of sourdough be the pelting brain? This, along whose busy circuitry run Reason and Madness in perpetual race—a race that most often ends in a tie? But the look deceives. What seems a fattish snail drowzing in its shell, in fact lives in quickness, where all is dart and stir and rapids of electricity.

Once again to the operating room.

How to cut a paste that is less solid than cheese, Brie, perhaps? And not waste any of it? For that would be a decade of remembrances and wishes lost there, wiped from the knife. Mostly it is done with cautery, burning the margins of the piece to be removed, coagulating with the fine electric current these blood vessels that course everywhere. First a spot is burned; then another alongside the first, and the cut is made between. One does not stitch—one cannot sew custard. Blood is blotted with little squares of absorbent gauze. These are called patties. Through each of these a long black thread has been sewn, lest a blood-soaked patty slip into some remote fissure, or flatten against a gyrus like a starfish against a coral reef, and go unnoticed come time to close the incision. A patty abandoned brainside benefits not the health, nor improves the climate of the intelligence. Like the bodies of slain warriors, they must be retrieved from the field, and carried home, in order that they not bloat and mortify, poisoning forever the plain upon which the battle was fought. One pulls them out by their black thread and counts them.

Listen to the neurosurgeon: "Patty, buzz, suck, cut," he says. Then, "Suck, cut, patty, buzz." It is as simple and as deadly as a nursery rhyme.

The surgeon knows the landscape of the brain, yet does not know how a thought is made. Do a billion fireflies skitter and wink? Do some then gather into a ball, pinch off from the core, and whorl way to expression in the free air? Man has grown envious of this mystery. He would master and subdue it electronically. He would construct a computer to rival or surpass the brain. He would harness Europa's bull to a plow. There are men who implant electrodes into the brain, that part where anger is kept. The rage center, they call it. They press a button, and a furious bull halts in midcharge, and lopes amiably to nuzzle his matador. Anger has turned to sweet compliance. Others sever whole tracts of brain cells with their knives, to mollify the insane. Here is surgery grown violent as rape. These men cannot know the brain. They have not the heart for it.

I last saw the brain in the emergency room. I wiped it from the shoulder of a young girl to make her smashed body more presentable to her father. Now I stand with him by the stretcher. We are arm in arm, like brothers. All at once there is that terrible silence of discovery. I glance at him—follow his gaze—and see that there is more brain upon her shoulder, newly slipped from the cracked skull. He bends forward a bit. He must make certain. It *is* her brain! I watch the knowledge expand upon his face, his face, so like hers. Smashed, too, in a different way. I, too, stare at the fragment flung wetly, now drying beneath the bright lights of the emergency room, its cargo of thoughts evaporating from it, mingling for this little time with his, with mine, before dispersing in the air.

On the east coast of the Argolid, in the northern part of the Peloponnese, lies Epidauros. O bury my heart there, in that place I have never seen, but that I love as a farmer loves his home soil. In a valley nearby, in the fourth century B.C., there was built the temple of Asklepios, the god of medicine. To a great open, colonnaded room, the abaton, came the sick from all over Greece. Here they lay down on pallets. As night fell, the priests, bearing fire for the lamps, walked among them, commanding them to sleep. They were told to dream of the god, and that he would come to them in their sleep in the form of a serpent, and that he would heal them. In the morning they arose cured. Walk the length of the abaton; the sick are in their places, each upon his pallet. Here is one that cannot sleep. See how his breath rises and falls against some burden that presses against it. At last, he dozes, only to awaken minutes later, unrefreshed. It is toward dawn. The night lamps flicker low, casting snaky patterns across the colonnade. Already the chattering swallows swoop in and out among the pillars. All at once the fitful eyes of the man cease their roving, for he sees between the candle-lamp and the wall the shadow of an upraised serpent, a great yellow snake with topaz eyes. It slides closer. It is arched and godlike. It bends above him, swaying, the tongue and the lamplight flickering as one. Exultant, he raises himself upon one arm, and with the other, reaches out for the touch that heals.

Here is the highest realization of the medical art. At Epidauros, no need for the workaday butchery I do. A man, already made separate by his disease, further withdraws from mankind by entering his dreams, surrendering to their power. It is an encounter with the divine in the natural miracle of healing. At Epidauros each healing was an epiphany of the gods. The physician who feels the divinity of his art will own the intuition to take part in the mystery of healing. Through such a doctor, out of the most prosaic of materials, herbs and tools, will a great beauty be born. Each time it is a transcendence of Nature into Art.

On the bulletin board in the front hall of the hospital where I work, there appeared a small white card of announcement. "Yeshi Dhonden," it read, "will make Rounds at six o'clock in the morning of June tenth." The particularities of the meeting were then given, followed by a notation at the end: "Yeshi Dhonden is Personal Physician to the Dalai Lama." I am not so leathery a skeptic that I would knowingly ignore an emissary from the gods. Not only might such sangfroid be inimical to one's earthly well-being, it could take care of eternity as well. Thus, on the morning of June tenth, I join the clutch of whitecoats waiting in the small conference room adjacent to the ward selected for the Rounds. The air in the room is heavy with ill-concealed dubiety, and suspicion of bamboozlement. At precisely six o'clock, he materializes, a short, golden, barrelly man dressed in a sleeveless robe of saffron and maroon. His scalp is shaven, and the only visible hair is a scanty black line above each hooded eye. Such a presence as befits the consort of a god.

He bows in greeting while his young interpreter makes the introduction. Yeshi Dhonden, we are told, will examine a patient selected by a member of the staff. The diagnosis is as unknown to Yeshi Dhonden as it is to us. The examination of the patient will take place in our presence, after which we will reconvene in the conference room where Yeshi Dhonden will discuss the case. We are further informed that, for two hours prior to the Rounds, Yeshi Dhonden has purified himself by bathing, fasting, and prayer. I, having breakfasted well, performed only the most desultory of ablutions, and given no thought at all to my soul, glance furtively at my fellows. What a soiled, uncouth lot we seem.

The patient had been awakened early, told that she was to be examined by a foreign doctor, and requested to produce a fresh specimen of urine. So that when we enter her room, the woman shows no surprise. She has long ago taken on that mixture of compliance and resignation that is the facies of chronic illness. This was to be but another in an endless series of tests and examinations. Yeshi Dhonden steps to the bedside while the rest stand apart, watching. For a long time he gazes at the woman, favoring no part of her body with his eyes, but seeming to fix his glance at a place just above her supine form. I, too, study her. No physical sign, nor obvious symptom gives clue as to the nature of her disease.

At last, he takes her by the hand, raising it in both of his own. Now he bends over the bed in a kind of crouching stance, his head drawn down into the collar of his robe. His eyes are closed as he feels for her pulse. In a moment he has found the

spot, and for the next half an hour, he remains thus, suspended above the patient like some exotic bird with folded
golden wings, holding the pulse of the woman beneath his fingers, cradling her hand in his. All the power of the man seems
to have been drawn down into this one purpose. It is palpation
of the pulse raised to the state of ritual. From the foot of the
bed where I stand, it is as though he and the patient have entered a special place of isolation, of apartness, about which
a vacancy hovers, and across which no violation is possible.
After a moment the woman rests back upon her pillow. From
time to time, she raises her head to look at the strange figure
pendant above her, then sinks back once more. I cannot see
their hands joined in a correspondence that is exclusive, inti-
mate, his fingertips receiving the voice of her sick body through
the rhythm and throb she offers at her wrist. All at once I am
envious, not of him, not of Yeshi Dhonden for his gift of
beauty and hóliness, but of her. I want to be held like that,
touched so, *received*. And there, in that familiar place, where I
am used to do my work, which is his work, I feel the kind of
love that some men equate with love of God. I know also that
I, who have palpated a hundred thousand pulses, have not felt
a single one—not truly.

At last, Yeshi Dhonden straightens, gently places the woman's
hand upon the bed, and steps back. The interpreter produces a
small wooden bowl and two sticks. Yeshi Dhonden pours a
portion of the urine specimen into the bowl, and proceeds to
whip the liquid with the two sticks. This he does for several
minutes until a foam is raised. Then, bowing above the bowl,
he inhales the odor three times. He sets down the bowl and
turns to leave. All this while, he has not uttered a single word.
As he nears the door, the woman raises her head and calls out
to him in a voice at once urgent and serene. "Thank you, Doctor," she says, and touches with her other hand the place he
had held on her wrist, as though to recapture something that
had visited there, a bird, a breeze. Yeshi Dhonden turns back
for a moment to gaze at her, then steps into the corridor.
Rounds are at an end.

We are seated once more in the conference room. Yeshi
Dhonden speaks now for the first time. Soft Tibetan sounds
that I have never heard before. He has barely begun when the

young interpreter begins to translate, the two voices continuing in tandem—a bilingual fugue, the one chasing the other. It is like the chanting of monks. He speaks of winds coursing through the body of the woman, currents that break against barriers, eddying. These vortices are in her blood, he says. The last spendings of an imperfect heart. Between the chambers of her heart, long, long before she was born, a wind had come, and blown open a deep gate that must never be opened. Through it charge the full waters of her river, as the mountain stream cascades in the springtime, battering, knocking loose the land, and flooding her breath. Thus he speaks, and is silent.

"May we now have the diagnosis?" a professor asks.

The host of these Rounds, the man who knows, answers:

"Congenital Heart Disease," he says. "Interventricular Septal Defect, with resultant Heart Failure."

A gateway in the heart, I think. That must not be opened. Through it charge the full waters that flood her breath. So! Here then is the doctor listening to the sounds of the body to which the rest of us are deaf. He is more than doctor. He is priest.

I know—I know—the doctor to the gods is pure knowledge, pure healing. The doctor to Man stumbles, must often wound; his patient must die, as must he. Still, now and then it happens as I make my own Rounds, that I hear the sounds of his voice, like an ancient Buddhist prayer, its meaning long since forgotten, only the music remaining. Then a jubilation possesses me, and I feel myself touched by something divine.

ALL   (*or almost all*)   Excellent! Bravo! (*applause*).

DICK SELZER   I have been attempting, as you see, to write about medicine and surgery, in the only way I can, to give it a meaning that is not obvious. As someone said this afternoon, the ordinary can become significant if it is gazed upon with a special look. But let's carry on.

BILL OBER   You know, pathologists are gadflies. Dick, what was your diagnosis for that skin lesion on the scalp?

DICK SELZER   That it was an epidermal carcinoma. Why?

BILL OBER   Oh. I just wondered. It might have been a kerato-acanthoma which heals itself in six months and looks exactly like a squamous carcinoma clinically and very much like one microscopically.

DICK SELZER   No good will ever come of you for having said that.

DENISE LEVERTOV   A tinker's curse!

DICK SELZER   Exactly. But this was based on a true story. And it *was* a carcinoma. I have the pathology to prove it.

BILL OBER   Uh-huh. That is one of the saddest mistakes made in medicine. I am very serious about this. I'm sorry to be an s.o.b. about it, but this is my business.

DICK SELZER   It doesn't change my diagnosis (but this is all so superficial as to be trivial). I prefer to think of the lesion as a cancer because it serves my purpose in this instance.

BILL OBER   It serves *my* purpose to point out that it might have been a keratoacanthoma, which is benign.

DICK SELZER   You're perfectly within your rights to respond to my writing any way you want. It's just that I—

GENE MOSS   Now just a minute! What that lesion was matters enormously in some ways, and in some ways it doesn't matter at all. What we are working on is "the healing arts," and it is from that artistic point of view that it doesn't matter.

NANCY ANDREASEN   If I had to choose between the knife and the holy water, much as I hate the knife, I'd choose it over the holy water any day.

GENE MOSS   Of course. But that's irrelevant too.

NANCY ANDREASEN   No, that's the moral impact of what Dick has written; that there is something holier than the mundane physical forms of treatment that we have available.

DICK SELZER   I find myself in a very peculiar position.

DENISE LEVERTOV   You are hearing an embattled panic against the very idea that the unexplainable or "supernatural" might exist.

NANCY ANDREASEN   On the contrary, I've gone on record as believing in the supernatural.

IAN LAWSON   Dick's description of the lesion was in words of truth. What the slide actually shows cannot alter that truthfulness. I think the description was beautiful.

ELIZABETH SEWELL   "Beauty is truth, truth, beauty."

BILL OBER   It can also be beautiful and true and dead wrong.

IAN LAWSON   It's not that it's "wrong." It's a matter of supplementary evidence. You can revise the histological diagnosis, but that's another dimension of truth.

GENE MOSS   We have a story, the primary responsibility of which is that it be faithful to language and to the medium in which it works. In the same way, the critic must be faithful to the literature with which he is working; the pathologist must be faithful to the organism with which he is working. If either of them fails, he is irresponsible. But we can't take the responsibility of the one and transfer it to the other.

BILL OBER   Yes, you can, and I do it every day in writing psychological biographies of writers.

GENE MOSS   I am not challenging the validity of what you do, but we have an art form in front of us and as critics, we have to be responsible to it.

DICK SELZER   I am shocked that this is the mode of discussion, though I should be accustomed to being misread.

BILL OBER   You're not being misread—you're being revised. What you've written is very beautiful and very good and I like it. But the question remains as to what you are dealing with in fact. Your story is true insofar as clinical observation goes. But there is another level of truth; that is, WHAT THE HELL IS IT?—And that can only be decided by somebody's observations with a microscope.

DICK SELZER   Have you never seen a miracle in all your years of medical practice?

BILL OBER   No!

ELIZABETH SEWELL   Bill, I can hear what you're saying, and I respect it, but, Dick, we shouldn't be talking to you this way. Your story was just beautiful.

JO TRAUTMANN   Let's break up for a while and go away. Those of us who want to can come back for more talk. (*Thirty minutes later*) Well, what happened?

IAN LAWSON   You may not believe it, but this amount of tension is quite normal in medical dialogue. This is the way pathologists and clinicians interact professionally. Medical practitioners—doctors, nurses, other health professionals—have very different views of the body. There is no single medical model, really. Dick, for instance, has quite a different perspective on the body than I have because of his practice. It's intrusive, respectful but intrusive. It lands more often inside body cavities, which I rarely view. In our practices, Nancy and I might only be able to prove our initial observations after months or years of care. So even if this were a pathological conference, that slide would probably be creating dissension among the pathologists.

GENE MOSS   It strikes me that something else is at work here. And it doesn't particularly come from the medical side, but rather from the literature side. One of the things which Dick's story expresses and captures so well for me at least is a kind of reverence for the art (of surgery) and the object of the art (the body), a reverence which professional literati feel regularly in their handling of literature. That triggers a whole set of reactions in me, not only in regard to the art work and the dignity, the correctness, with which it must be treated, but also a reverence for the way in which the story is rendered artistically. In dealing with ailments of the body, we've got to be damned disciplined and correct scientifically in every way possible. But my expectation is that in our medical students we would inculcate some reverence for that dimension of life which cannot be known fully through an examination of a slide.

JO TRAUTMANN   Bill, to clarify these tensions further, may I ask you what you do with the aspects of life which you cannot find in your microscope?

BILL OBER These do not appear in a pathologist's report.

JO TRAUTMANN I know, but I mean you, as a person, as a whole human being. Or do you live your life as a pathologist *and*—as Bill Ober?

BILL OBER Oh, there is an enormous dichotomy. There are things you do professionally, paying no attention to the quality of life but strict attention to the facts as observed.

JO TRAUTMANN Do you do that without devotion?

BILL OBER We do it carefully and well and according to the canons of our trade.

JO TRAUTMANN Isn't there a certain beauty in that?

BILL OBER There is nothing beautiful in passing death sentences.

JIM COWAN I think what has happened really isn't about Dick's story at all, though it was the immediate catalyst. I think something has been going on since the first meeting, although I wasn't conscious of it then because I was caught up in my own wish-fulfillment fantasies about dialogues. Basically, there are two totally different world views at work. One approach is quantitative and analytical in its inherent value, and the other is likely to value intuition, perceptions, nuances of feeling in art, and so on.

DENISE LEVERTOV That may be true at the extremes. But in fact most of what goes on in this group is in the middle, including those places where they overlap.

NANCY ANDREASEN I too would really hate to see the group disintegrate into two competing schools because I don't think that's really the case. I have enormous respect for the intuitive mode. I can't use it most of the time in treating patients. I can sometimes because I am a psychiatrist. But if I were a surgeon—

DICK SELZER But intuition is the most important thing I use! That surprises you? It surprises me too. I can only say that I could never do this thing I do again if I did not feel I could bring to it all the intuition I have.

NANCY ANDREASEN Reverence is what you have, not intuition. Where you cut is based on science, not intuition.

DICK SELZER I disagree with that, Nancy. And it is the reason I write. Otherwise I would mind my own business. This intuition is the mark of a great doctor. Speaking for myself, I don't think it's possible to separate science from intuition.

NANCY ANDREASEN You know, Ian was saying at dinner that to understand the problems of dealing with patients, you have to go in and see them. And when Dick was reading, I was thinking, "I wish someone like Denise or Elizabeth could have the same physical feeling that Dick is able to have in touching human organs."

DICK SELZER I think Denise and Elizabeth understand perfectly.

DENISE LEVERTOV As poets, Elizabeth and I are in the habit of touching daily in our imaginations more things than a lot of people do in one year. I don't mean to sound boastful. It's simply part of our trade.

NANCY ANDREASEN That's one of the differences between the two trades. Medical people have to go in and touch something with their hands in order to believe it, while poetic people can project towards it with their imaginations.

ELIZABETH SEWELL Can I say something about polarities? We're setting up two poles, because we're trained to think of them that way, as oppositions. But with some poets and philosophers, each pole is the precondition of the other.

DENISE LEVERTOV Imagine a glistening, gleaming thread between two poles. The poles are then cooperating in upholding a lovely tension between them.

IAN LAWSON No, no, what you're facing is the effect that the phenomenon of illness has on those of us who have to live with it. And I'm afraid that your poetic empathy will not take you into this dimension. An ill person is not a normal person less something. There is very little you can do to prepare yourself to deal with illness, particularly morbid illness, because it is a unique human activity.

BILL OBER   Two different perspectives, but I believe this gap can be bridged. May I give you a preview of coming attractions? Jim's paper on D. H. Lawrence is the one scheduled for discussion tomorrow. It is just the sort I would love to present to a group of medical students because it is creative and constructive literary criticism. People are at liberty to disagree with Lawrence's view of anatomy. But not with Jim's exposition of it.

DICK SELZER   I'm looking forward to discussing your paper.

JIM COWAN   I'm not.

18 October 1975

D. H. LAWRENCE AND THE RESURRECTION OF THE BODY
James C. Cowan

"I believe in the resurrection of the body," Lady Constance Chatterley says (*LCL*, p. 98),[8] and she means it rather literally in the here and now. D. H. Lawrence uses the Christian mystery of resurrection as a profound symbol of the emergence into living sensuality which he wanted to see humanity make in his time from the torpor, indeed the death and putrefaction, of an overintellectualized established religion that supported the economic and social status quo of an industrial society that turned people of flesh and blood into machines.

T. S. Eliot's Prufrock, though so far as I know in normal health physically, had experienced this death-in-life state as the walking zombie of the room where "the women come and go/Talking of Michaelangelo," whose magnificent masculine figures stand in sharp contrast to Prufrock's physique, with its thinning hair and thinner arms and legs. In the opening lines of "The Love Song of J. Alfred Prufrock," as Stephen Spender suggests, Prufrock projects his condition outward upon the landscape in the simile of the "patient etherised upon a table," an image unsuitable to describe an evening but singularly accurate in characterizing Prufrock and his anaesthetized society.[9] As Spender points out, Lawrence, rather than projecting modern man's torpor upon the natural environment, internalizes nature itself as a resurrective principle:[10]

A sun will rise in me,
I shall slowly resurrect,
already the whiteness of false dawn is on my inner ocean.

(*CP*, p. 513)

In his review of Tolstoi's *Resurrection*, Lawrence declares: "We have all this time been worshipping a dead Christ: or a dying." Christians should know better: "The Cross was only the first step into achievement. The second step was the tomb. And the third step, whither?" In Tolstoi, he felt, "the stone was rolled upon him" (*P*, p. 737), leaving Christ a God of death and spirit, not of life and flesh. In "The Risen Lord," Lawrence claims that "the Churches insist on Christ Crucified, and rob us of the fruit of the year," for in the liturgical calendar, all the months from Easter to Advent belong to "the risen Lord" (*P*, p. 571). For Lawrence, "resurrection of the body" meant, in part, "resurrection of the flesh":

> If Jesus rose from the dead in triumph, a man on earth triumphant in renewed flesh, triumphant over the mechanical anti-life convention of Jewish priests, Roman despotism, and universal money-lust; triumphant above all over His own self-absorption, self-consciousness, self-importance; triumphant and free as a man in full flesh and full, final experience, even the accomplished acceptance of His own death; a man at last full and free in flesh and soul, a man at one with death: then He rose to become at one with life, to live the great life of the flesh and the soul together, as peonies or foxes do, in their lesser way. If Jesus rose as a full man, in full flesh and soul, then He rose to take a woman to Himself, to live with her, and to know the tenderness and blossoming of the twoness with her; He who had been hitherto so limited to His oneness, or His universality, which is the same thing. (*P II*, p. 575)

Lawrence's theology perhaps owes something to the medieval Adamites, who sought to return man to the state of innocence before the Fall; or at least to Joachim of Flora, the thirteenth-century abbot, whose division of history into the epoch of the Father before Christ, the epoch of the Son from the Advent of Christ to the present, and the epoch of the Holy Ghost yet to come Lawrence had cited favorably in *Movements in European History* (*MEH*, pp. 193–94).

Without elaborating further on Lawrence's theological position, I want to suggest that "the risen Lord" throughout his canon, particularly in his later work, is a paradigm for a resurgence of the flesh and the deep, intuitive knowledge available to man through sensual awareness as equal in value to the mind and the mental-spiritual knowledge elevated by the Protestant-capitalist-materialist ethos of modern industrial society. If the emphasis in Western culture upon rational, objective knowledge validated in the laboratory may be seen as the masculine thrust of spirit, the externalization of Idea in the technological penetration, control, and exploitation of nature, from the smallest organism to the moon and stars, in the quest for immutable scientific law, then Lawrence's reaffirmation of intuitive, subjective knowledge validated experientially in the body is an attempt to redeem the feminine, the inward, the mutable as a significant mode of knowing lost to whole generations immured in the scientific method.

Lawrence's treatment of physicians is not kind—when they lend their skills in the once priestly art of medicine to the warfare state in conducting pre-induction physical examinations. In *Kangaroo* the first examining physicians encountered by Lawrence's persona, Somers, address him as one gentleman to another and reject the thin, apparently consumptive man for military service (*K*, p. 233). At a later stage in the war, when almost no one is being rejected, the doctors at the induction center treat him in far less gentlemanly fashion. They are contemptuous of his body, Somers feels, and sneeringly skeptical when he tells them he has had pneumonia three times and is threatened with consumption. He submits in silent rage as they examine his genitals and rectum. "Never again," he vows to himself, "never would he be touched again. And because they had handled his private parts, and looked into them, their eyes should burst and their hands should wither and their hearts should rot. So he cursed them in his blood . . ." (*K*, p. 261). And why? Why should Lawrence recoil from the same kind of physical examination which millions of men have undergone for military service? Lawrence's own neurotic motives aside, he recoils not from another's touching his body but from the body's being objectified, reduced to a static part in an inexorable mechanism for killing in a world without grace, rather than being treated reverently as subject and human, functional in an organic and holy world. Somers is not the German spy his Cornish neighbors accuse him of being; his subversion goes much deeper than that: "This trench and machine warfare is a blasphemy against life itself, a blasphemy which we are all committing" (*K*, p. 225).

In such a world, touch is violation. As Lawrence puts it in "Touch," a poem from *Pansies*:

Since we are so cerebral
we are humanly out of touch.
And so we must remain.
For if, cerebrally, we force ourselves into touch,
   into contact
physical and fleshly,
we violate ourselves,
we become vicious.

(*CP*, p. 468)

A basic tenet of Lawrence's thinking is that sensory or sensual experience should not be dominated by ideas or ideals mentally derived. Hence his pronouncements against "sex in the head" and his cry in another poem from *Pansies*:

Noli me tangere, touch me not.
O you creatures of mind, don't touch me!
O you with mental fingers, O never put your hand on me!
O you with mental bodies, stay a little distance from me!

(*CP*, p. 468)

And hence, in a third poem in the sequence, his call for "Chastity, beloved chastity" in "this mind-mischievous age":

O leave me clean from mental fingering
from the cold copulation of the will,
from all the white self-conscious lechery
the modern mind calls love!

$(CP,$ p. 469$)$

The alternative, in our age, as he suggests in a fourth poem in
the sequence, is a resurrection of touch in the very blood:

Touch comes when the white mind sleeps
and only then.
Touch comes slowly, if ever; it seeps
slowly up in the blood of men
and women.

Soft slow sympathy
of the blood in me, of the blood in thee
rises and flushes insidiously
over the conscious personality
of each of us. . . .

Personalities exist apart;
and personal intimacy has no heart.
Touch is of the blood
uncontaminated, the unmental flood.

$(CP,$ pp. 470–71$)$

There was an age, Lawrence postulates in *Etruscan Places*,
when touch had the nonmental yet sacramental quality he
wants. In describing the wall paintings in the *Tomba dei Vasi
Dipinti* (Tomb of the Painted Vases), Lawrence remarks on
the banquet scene with "the bearded man softly touching the
woman with him under the chin":

Rather gentle and lovely is the way he touches the woman
under the chin, with a delicate caress. That again is one of the
charms of the Etruscan paintings: they really have the sense of
touch; the people and the creatures are all really in touch. It is
one of the rarest qualities, in life as well as in art. There is
plenty of pawing and laying hold, but no real touch. In pictures especially, the people may be in contact, embracing or
laying hands on one another. But there is no soft flow of

touch. The touch does not come from the middle of the human being. It is merely a contact of surfaces, and a juxtaposition of objects. . . . Here, in this faded Etruscan painting, there is a quiet flow of touch that unites the man and the woman on the couch, the timid boy behind, the dog that lifts his nose, even the very garlands that hang from the wall. (*EP*, pp. 77–78)

So it seems to Lawrence because he envisions ancient Etruria as a civilization whose knowledge emerged from integrated physical, intellectual, and emotional being instead of compartmentalizing both knowledge and being into so many intersecting surfaces and manipulatable fragments:

It must have been a wonderful world, that old world where everything appeared alive and shining in the dusk of contact with all things, not merely as an isolated individual thing played upon by daylight; where each thing had a clear outline, visually, but in its very clarity was related emotionally or vitally to strange other things, one thing springing from another, things mentally contradictory fusing together emotionally. (*EP*, pp. 112–13)

This vitalistic philosophy was rooted in a nonanthropomorphic religion whose gods "were not *beings*, but symbols of elemental powers": "The undivided Godhead, if we can call it such, was symbolised by the *mundum*, the plasm-cell with its nucleus: that which is the very beginning, instead of, as with us, by a personal god, a person being the very end of all creation or evolution" (*EP*, p. 87).

The *mundum* as plasm-cell is the central metaphor for man in the psychological theory which Lawrence elaborates in *Psychoanalysis and the Unconscious* and *Fantasia of the Unconscious*. In Lawrence's mythic metaphor, "The original nucleus, formed from the two parent nuclei at our conception, remains always primal and central, and is always the original fount and knowledge that *I am I*" (*FU*, p. 75). As the first of four dynamic psychic centers in what Lawrence calls "the first field of consciousness," this center remains "within the solar plexus" as the medium of a sympathetic, positive mode of knowing by incorporating the outer world into the self. Through this medium, in vital polarity with the mother's solar plexus, the infant maintains a pure, effluent, preverbal communication with her. Individuation occurs as the original nucleus divides (though paradoxically Lawrence suggests, in contradiction of the principle of cell division, that it remains in the solar plexus): "This second nucleus, the nucleus born of recoil, is the nuclear origin of all the great nuclei of the voluntary system, which are the nuclei of assertive individualism" (*FU*, p. 76). In the adult, this second center remains in what Lawrence calls "the lumbar ganglion" as a subjective medium of differentiation and negativity: "*I am myself, and these others are not as I am*" (*FU*, p. 79). The third and fourth centers emerge as the first two divide horizontally. Whereas the centers of the lower dynamic plane are subjective in nature, those of the upper dynamic plane are objective, and upper and lower are supposed to complement each other (*PU*, p. 34). The cardiac plexus has the same relation to the thoracic ganglion that the solar plexus has to the lumbar ganglion. Like the solar plexus, the cardiac plexus is positive and sympathetic, but rather than incorporating the other into the self, it sees in the other an object of worship in which to lose the self: "The wonder is without me. . . . The other being is now the great positive reality, I myself am as nothing" (*FU*, p. 78). The thoracic ganglion, like the lumbar ganglion, is negative in polarity, but whereas the lumbar ganglion functions instinctually, for example in expressing rage, the thoracic ganglion is the seat of the spiritual will whereby one manipulates others. In harmonious balance with the lower centers, the upper centers serve useful functions. The thoracic ganglion becomes the source of "eager curiosity, of the delightful desire to pick things to pieces, and the desire to put them together again, the desire to 'find out,' and the desire to invent. . . ." (*FU*, p. 80). In the integrated individual, Lawrence suggests, not only do the four dynamic psychic centers function harmoniously together but also they function in balanced polarity with the psychic centers of the other in a human relationship.

In May 1918, Lawrence wrote to Edith Eder, the wife of Dr. David Eder and the sister of Barbara Low, both of them London psychoanalysts, asking her to find him a book on the human nervous system with maps. Had she referred him to a standard medical text such as Gray's *Anatomy of the Human Body*, then available in the twentieth edition revised, edited by Warren H. Lewis (Philadelphia: Lea and Febiger, 1918), pages 701–21, he would have found a scientific exposition of the two broad divisions of the human nervous system into the central nervous system, the brain and spinal cord, and the peripheral nervous system, composed of the voluntary nervous system, which mediates voluntary movements, and the autonomic, or as Lewis's edition of Gray calls it, the sympathetic nervous system, which mediates involuntary physical functions of the glands, blood vessels, and the like.

But Lawrence, while sometimes claiming scientific validity and sometimes admitting to scientific inexactitude, "particularly in terminology" (*FU*, p. 36), makes no claim to objective scientific knowledge based on the doctrine of logical positivism, which limits science to what can be deduced by rigorous logic from the observation and classification of factual data and sensory phenomena. Rather he posited a "subjective science," as he called it, derived from the ancients, from the vitalists and the animists, from the Etruscans and the Egyptians; a science of intuition and imagination rather than of cause and effect; a science in which poet and healer are not separate, as in the modern world, but the same, as in the poet-priest-king-medicine man tradition.

Lawrence's "science" is that of a poet. He wrote: "This pseudophilosophy of mine—'pollyanalytics,' as one of my respected critics might say—is deduced from the novels and poems, not the reverse" (*FU*, p. 57). Even so, he does not proceed deductively but declares: "I proceed by intuition" (*FU*, p. 54). And the system he proposes is not based on objective fact but on metaphor. His four dynamic psychic centers are all parts of the autonomic nervous system, transmitting impulses and mediating involuntary functions, not, as he seems to suggest, the great integrative centers, which modern neuroanatomy locates in the central nervous system, of such complex functions as integration, origin of impulses, and consciousness. So what is the value of a metaphor rooted in inaccuracy or of a nonscientific science? For Lawrence the value lies in formulating a personal myth to affirm what the body knows as opposed to what the mind knows. Implicit in his theory is the criticism that in the modern world the upper centers of mind and spirit have gained the upper hand while the lower centers of body and blood have declined. The will dominates; instinct atrophies.

To resurrect the science of the ancients, then, is to resurrect the body. That is what Lawrence undertakes imaginatively in *Lady Chatterley's Lover*. From the beginning of her marriage, Lady Constance Chatterley had wanted children, but at that time she had thought that "sex was merely an accident, or an adjunct, one of the curious, obsolete, organic processes which persisted in its own clumsiness, but was not really necessary" (*LCL*, p. 11). Now as Sir Clifford, who has returned from the war paralyzed from the waist down, sits with his friends in long, intellectual conversation, she muses on their curious one-sidedness: "How many evenings had Connie sat and listened to the manifestations of these four men: . . . It was fun. Instead of kissing you, and touching you, they revealed their minds to you. It was great fun! But what cold minds" (*LCL*, p.39). Formulating a vague plan to have a child, she recalls the biblical text, "Go ye into the streets and byways of Jerusalem and see if you can find *a man*" (*LCL*, p. 73). The relationship might even be impersonal if forces greater than their social selves were present. Shortly after this Connie comes upon Mellors, the gamekeeper, bathing in the back yard of his cottage:

> He was naked to the hips, his velveteen breeches slipping down over his slender loins. And his white slim back was curved over a big bowl of soapy water, in which he ducked his head, shaking his head with a queer, quick little motion, lifting his slender white arms, and pressing the soapy water from his ears, quick, subtle as a weasel playing with water, and utterly alone. (*LCL*, p. 75)

This scene, which resembles closely the bathing girl scene at the end of chapter 4 of James Joyce's *A Portrait of the Artist as a Young Man*, recounts an experience as remarkable as Stephen's epiphany of dovelike female beauty, yet this is an epiphany, as it were, of the solar plexus, not of the mind:

> In spite of herself, she had had a shock. After all, merely a man washing himself; commonplace enough, Heaven knows! Yet in some curious way it was a visionary experience: it

had hit her in the middle of her body. She saw the clumsy breeches slipping down over the pure, delicate, white loins, the bones showing a little, and the sense of aloneness, of a creature purely alone, overwhelmed her. Perfect, white, solitary nudity of a creature that lives alone, and inwardly alone. And beyond that, a certain beauty of a pure creature. Not the stuff of beauty, not even the body of beauty, but a lambency, the warm, white flame of a single life, revealing itself in contours that one might touch: a body!

Connie had received the shock of vision in her womb, and she knew it; it lay inside her. (*LCL*, p. 76)

That evening, looking at her own body in the mirror, Connie thinks, "What a frail, easily hurt, rather pathetic thing a human body is, naked; somehow a little unfinished, incomplete!" (*LCL*, p. 79). She sees that, "instead of ripening its firm, down-running curves, her body was flattening and going a little harsh. It was as if it had not had enough sun and warmth; it was a little grayish and sapless" (*LCL*, p. 80). Deprived of its very existence, "her body was going meaningless, going full and opaque, so much insignificant substance" (*LCL*, p. 80). Tommy Dukes, who seems at times to deliver Lawrence's own criticism of his society and his age, confirms Connie's judgment of their bodiless and meaningless existence, but looks to the future: "There might even be real men, in the next phase. . . . *We're* not men, and the women aren't women. We're only cerebrating makeshifts, mechanical and intellectual experiments" (*LCL*, p. 86).

What is it that stands between Connie Chatterley and the life of her own body? Lawrence suggests that it is mental life, the habit of living from the mind alone instead of the vital centers of the body, or, worse, the motivating of these centers of spontaneous instinct by ideas: "How she hated words, always coming between her and life: they did the ravishing, if anything did: ready made words and phrases" (*LCL*, p. 108).

Yet opposed to the world of words, Sir Clifford Chatterley's trivial if fashionably witty writing and conversation, the intellectual counterpart of his mining industry, is the world of organic nature, the forest preserve of the old England on which the mines encroach further and further. Connie's second epiphany of the body comes at the gamekeeper's hut as she watches a pheasant chick, which has just emerged from the *mundum* of the egg, bravely asserting its identity to the universe: ". . . it was the most alive little spark of a creature in seven kingdoms at that moment. Connie crouched to watch in a sort of ecstasy. Life, life! Pure, sparky, fearless new life! New life! So tiny and so utterly without fear!" (*LCL*, p. 133). Mellors gives her a chick to hold:

> She took the little drab thing between her hands, and there it stood, on its impossible little stalks of legs, its atom of balancing life trembling through its almost weightless feet into Connie's hands. But it lifted its handsome, clean-shaped little head boldly, and looked sharply round, and gave a little "peep."
> "So adorable! So cheeky!" she said softly.
> The keeper, squatting beside her, was also watching with an amused face the bold little bird in her hands. Suddenly he saw a tear fall on to her wrist. (*LCL*, p. 135)

The resurrection of the flesh begins almost immediately as Mellors, who in his taciturn disappointment in marriage had thought the sexual life was finished for him, feels "the old flame shooting and leaping up in his loins, that he had hoped was quiescent for ever" (*LCL*, p. 135). The two make love in the hut on an army blanket on the floor. Connie lies as if in a dream:

> The activity, the orgasm was his, all his; she could strive for herself no more. Even the tightness of his arm round her, even the intense movement of his body, and the springing seed in her, was a kind of sleep, from which she did not begin to rouse till he had finished and lay softly panting against her breast. (*LCL*, p. 137)

Feminist critics like Kate Millett have deplored Connie's passivity[11] and missed the genuine tenderness of Mellors's regard for her. I do not think that Lawrence sees himself as writing a poetic marriage manual any more than I think that his direct description of sexual acts in the novel tends to deprave and corrupt. Lawrence is neither prescribing passivity for women nor titillating bourgeois men. I take Connie's sleeplike state as a symbolic death of her mental life presaging a resurrection of the body.

This rebirth is an evolution into life, developed gradually in the novel in the sexual experiences which Connie and Mellors share. For valid medical description of sexual data, phenomena observed and catalogued with scientific conclusions drawn from them, Masters's and Johnson's *Human Sexual Response* is, perhaps, more reliable than *Lady Chatterley's Lover*. But having said so, I am reminded that in *Human Sexual Inadequacy*, Masters and Johnson as sex therapists characteristically turn to the touch and tenderness that informed Lawrence's last major novel. Sir Clifford Chatterley, his lower centers literally paralyzed, rolls over the flowers of the wood in his motorized wheel chair, a symbol for his whole mechanical being. Connie and Mellors, vulnerable but reborn, reject the single-minded life of surface mentality and the machine civilization that it serves. Hermits of love, as impractical as the love saints of John Donne's "The Canonization," they burn like tapers and rise in the flame like the phoenix, Lawrence's image of resurrection par excellence. "We fucked a flame into being," Mellors writes to Connie:

> You can't insure against the future, except by really believing in the best bit of you, and in the power behind it. So I believe in the little flame between us. . . . It's my Pentecost, the forked flame between me and you. . . . That's what I abide by, and will abide by, Cliffords and Berthas, colliery companies and governments and the money-mass of people all notwithstanding. (*LCL*, p. 364)

Although the civilization as a whole seems doomed, the "forked flame" of sexual tenderness and the baby Connie carries in her womb are symbols of the hope for individual love with which the novel ends.

The "resurrection of the body" becomes, finally, the central theme in the last novella Lawrence published in his lifetime, appearing in London under the title *The Man Who Died* but published first in Paris as *The Escaped Cock* (1929), titles which reflect opposing cultural emphases on death and rebirth. Although Lawrence clearly bases his story on biblical accounts of Christ's appearances after death, he does not identify the protagonist as Christ, because he has rejected His messianic mission, or Jesus, because that would restrict him to the historical Jesus, but simply as "the man," for the purpose of wholly humanizing and secularizing the figure by embodying in him the principle of life renewed in the flesh rather than in the spirit.

The essay "The Risen Lord," written in the same year, is an excellent gloss on the novella.

In another paper, I have demonstrated Lawrence's technique of making biblical allusions in a context which consistently alters the original heavenly or spiritual meaning to an earthly, physical one. For example, John's account of Christ's words to Mary Magdalene, "Touch me not; for I am not yet ascended to my Father: but go to my brethren, and say unto them, I ascend to my Father, and your Father; and to my God, and your God" (John 20:17), is revised in Lawrence's version to read, "Don't touch me, Madeleine. . . . Not yet! I am not yet healed and in touch with men" (*MWD*, p. 24), for the purpose of suggesting a shift in allegiance from the spiritual forces implied in ascending "to my Father" to the physical awareness of being "in touch with men." Lawrence had been hostile to John's doctrine of creation by the Logos (John 1:1) at least as far back as the unpublished Foreword to *Sons and Lovers*, which attempts to restore the primacy of flesh over word. Now the risen man concludes:

> The Word is but the midge that bites at evening. Man is tormented with words like midges, and they follow him right into the tomb. But beyond the tomb they cannot go. Now I have passed the place where words can bite no more and the air is clear, and there is nothing to say, and I am alone within my own skin, which is the walls of all my domain. (*MWD*, p. 38)

The Apostle Paul's definition of the meaning of the Resurrection is that "our Saviour Jesus Christ . . . hath abolished death, and hath brought life and immortality to light through the gospel" (2 Tim. 1:10), but Lawrence's risen man wants only to heal his wounds and enjoy "the immortality of being alive without fret. For in the tomb he had left his striving self . . ." (*MWD*, p. 39).

The escaped cock of Lawrence's title, an allusion to the cock that crowed after Peter's third denial of Christ on the night of his trial, refers literally to a gamecock which breaks his fetters at the same moment that the man awakens "from a long sleep in which he [has been] tied up" in the tomb, and figuratively, of course, to the phallus and the new vital life of the blood. Part 2 of the novella introduces the Isis-Osiris myth in the risen man's journey to the temple of Isis in Search, where he stays in a cave of goats, an obvious reference to Pan. Both his sepulchre, "a carved hole in the rock" (*MWD*, p. 7) and the cave, a dark place in which there is "a little basin of rock where the maidenhair fern [fringes] a dripping mouthful of water" (*MWD*, p. 62) are womb symbols. His emergence from the tomb marks his rebirth into physical life, but his emergence from the cave signals a rebirth of long repressed sexuality. When he goes to the priestess who identifies him with the lost Osiris, he admits to himself, "I am almost more afraid of this touch than I was of death. For I am more nakedly exposed to it" (*MWD*, p. 84). "It has hurt so much!" he says to her. "You must forgive me if I am held back." But the woman answers softly, "Let me anoint you! . . . Let me anoint the scars!" (*MWD*, pp. 87–88). Through this touch, he realizes why he had been put to death: "I had asked them to serve me with the corpse of their love. And in the end I offered them only the corpse of my love." But his followers could not love "with dead bodies," and he reflects, "If I had kissed Judas with a live love, perhaps he would never have kissed me with death" (*MWD*, pp. 89–90).

This new self-knowledge signals a growth in being that is inwardly organic: as in the poem "Sun in Me," "a new sun was coming up in him" (*MWD*, p. 93). Whereas Christ had built his church upon the rock of St. Peter (Matt. 16:18), the risen man, touching the woman, thinks, "On this rock I built my life" (*MWD*, p. 94). Having rejected the spiritual communion of the broken body that he had instituted earlier, he wants now only the sacrament of the communion of flesh with flesh. In a multi leveled pun that is, at once, an allusion to scriptural Resurrection (Luke 24:6) and a literalization in sexual terms of the Laurentian "resurrection of the body," the man says, at the very moment of phallic erection, "I am risen!" (*MWD*, p. 94). After their sexual consummation, he says, "This is the great atonement, the being in touch," for in the new life "atonement" means human relatedness that does not depend on the sacrifice of the divine pharmakos.

Nevertheless, Lawrence's risen man, though de-Christianized, is subtly mythicized through blending with the figure of Osiris. Both Osiris and Christ are associated with the miracle of wine both were betrayed by "brothers," slain, and deified. But Christ's Resurrection was followed by his Ascension, whereas Osiris, in the version of the myth that concerns Lawrence, did not, properly speaking, rise. Instead the goddess Isis went in search for the pieces of his body, which his evil brother Set had dismembered and scattered along the Nile, and she found all but the phallus. Lawrence so carefully fuses the two figures that his risen man, though based on the celibate Jesus, is made to supply what is missing in the Osiris myth. "Rare women," the philosopher has told the priestess of Isis in Search, "wait for the re-born man" (*MWD*, p. 58), and she is one of those rare women. Identified on the one hand with the Magna Mater archetype and on the other with the tradition of the sacred prostitute, she is presented primarily in terms of her priestly function of healing. Even her pregnancy is not treated realistically but, in keeping with the tone of solemnity appropriate to the quest romance, is linked with the fruition of the natural cycle of the seasons. The man, too, rather than ascending in a vertical, linear thrust of spirit like his biblical counterpart, identifies himself, like Osiris, with the seasonal cycle as he departs: "Be at peace. And when the nightingale calls again from your valley-bed, I shall come again, sure as Spring" (*MWD*, p. 100).

With hindsight, the first part of the dialogists' discussion of Jim Cowan's paper seems a cautious redoing of the debate on the previous evening. We were interested in establishing how far Lawrence strayed from the knowledge of anatomy he might have gained from Gray. It seemed important to almost everyone that as Jim worked on his projected edition of *Psychoanalysis and the Unconscious* and *Fantasia of the Unconscious*, he make some statement about Lawrence's accuracy. At the same time, most of us quite readily accepted Lawrence's organization of the body as a valuable metaphor, based to some extent upon actuality. We accepted him as, in his own terms, a "subjective scientist" and we pursued that label a little further. Some of us felt that Lawrence knew more about the body than many people in medicine, but that he came to his knowledge via a route that still seems unusual, at the very least. Quoting William Blake, Elizabeth Sewell reminded us that the nature of the visionary imagination is almost unknown.

The second part of the discussion derived from the question of how *Lady Chatterley's Lover* related to the importance of touch in medical situations. Dick Selzer maintained that as at Epidauros centuries earlier, a doctor's touch was part of the healing process. Ian Lawson agreed that touch heals, but through the more immediately explainable channels of rapport and tenderness, which should flow smoothly to investigative touch. To psychiatrist Nancy Andreasen, touch was another matter, though she is atypical because she does physical examinations on her patients.

The special situation for psychiatrists led the dialogists to consider the specifically sexual aspects of touch, directing the discussion back to Lawrence. Elizabeth noted that just as Dick had described in erotic terms the sort of surgery he did, so do many of us who teach enter the realm of the erotic when we touch our students. By implication she urged us not to be afraid of this part of our relationship with them. "Erotic," she said, had perhaps taken on too technical a meaning. In closing, Jo reminded the dialogists that even the technically erotic *Lady Chatterley's Lover* had once been entitled *Tenderness*; and that in the *Symposium* Eryximachus declares that medicine is a knowledge of the forces of Love in the body.

The Language of Medical Care
Imagination and Magic
Unities and Polarities

29 January 1976

Bill Ober did not come to Meeting Three, nor to the next one, because he was very ill. Nevertheless, the questions he had raised continued to demand our attention, beginning with Ian Lawson's paper on medical language. In turn, Ian provoked a poem from Denise Levertov and an essay from Jim Cowan, both of whom addressed the specter of the pathologist-poet split, but did not put it to rest. From Elizabeth Sewell we wanted to hear just what she proposed to resurrect when she spoke of "the other tradition." In an evening session even more remarkable than that evening in October, we may have found out.

THE PLACE OF LANGUAGE IN MEDICAL SCIENCE
AND PRACTICE

Ian Lawson

Our last meeting showed how far we could go in appearing to agree (because we wanted to and because words were coming well), but not in fact agreeing. Unexpected, but necessary therefore, was the rending of our rapport at the last meeting, not because one from the humanities turned on a physician, or vice versa, but because one physician turned on another.

Dick Selzer had written several sketches based obviously on

individual patient encounters in his practice. However, one of the cases implied miraculous cure. For that reason, the pathologist hunted down relentlessly the pathological details of the case, exposed an unsuspected ambiguity, destroyed the rapport, and generally confounded us. Nevertheless, after the discussion the consensus of the physicians (including the pursued author) was that the pathologist had done the right thing—right both by his assertion and by his obduracy. Why was he right? Because the scientific facts of a case are more important than its literary merit? That would imply that literary quality is an adornment, not an essential to medicine. Rather, in his pursuit to identify ambiguity (where reasonable certainty had been presumed), Bill Ober was reinforcing a major if less recognized function of language as well as a recognized function of science.

I think this event also suggested something about the physician writing qua physician (with or without the use of a pseudonym). For one thing, the physician has absolutely no poetic license, even if writing for a nonmedical audience. Vocabulary, syntax, style, content—all must be subject to the criteria of probability. With what certainty, probability, possibility, are the things stated likely to be so? There is no way he can divest himself of that burden of proof or of so underwriting his statements. To a medical audience, he will be required to show proof. Before a nonmedical audience, he will be assumed to have provided, or to be capable of providing, that proof to his peers.

This is not incompatible with good writing. But it means that such writing is subject to the professional obligations of the author.

The exploration and usage of verbal material is still the most important tool in the practice and science of medicine. It is not merely the communicative end product of a logical, mathematical process that has little use for it otherwise. Nor is it only a useful approximation or a shorthand for more complex symbolic forms (e.g., "the double helical" for the molecular architecture of DNA). It is still the principal stuff of patient-doctor interaction and of professional communication. It is also the medium of conceptualization, of making hypotheses, of inferring and deducing results, of summarizing and reducing masses of information to usable forms without deformity. It is the matrix in which thought and action cohere, even when quantification seems uppermost.

To say all this is not, on the other hand, to denigrate the place of measurement and calculation, or the place of mathematical and statistical models. Indeed, in several different ways modern mensuration and calculation have heightened (not replaced or diminished) the need for adequacy in the tools of language in medicine.

First, the "new mathematics" is insistent on the concurrent development of a logical use of word concepts, and of an ability to give the verbal correlates of mathematical statements. Alvan Feinstein has developed this double necessity in his text on "Clinical Judgment,"[1] utilizing the new mathematics to state a logic of inference that also requires a new "taxonomy of illness" in which to function:

"Clinical judgment depends not on a knowledge of causes, mechanisms, or names for disease, but on a knowledge of patients. The background of clinical judgment is clinical experience—the things clinicians have learned at bedside in the care of sick people. In acquiring this experience, every clinician has to use some sort of intellectual mechanism for organizing and remembering his observations." He continues:

"I had inadvertently worked out a rational description for at least a part of this intellectual mechanism. The system of clinical classification was a coherent, logical technique for cataloging the information used as a basis for clinical judgment. With that realization, I then rewrote and simplified my original paper on classification, emphasizing the value of Boolean algebra and clinical taxonomy in the clinical judgment with which doctors plan and appraise treatment."

Second, the computer has imposed rigid requirements of consistency as regards syntax and vocabulary. In so doing, the intolerance the machine has for ambiguity in its language has surely heightened our awareness of the remarkable place it has in human language. Here we are thinking of ambiguity not as carelessness or obscurity but as something attractive, preoccupying, enlightening in its indefinability.

Kenneth Burke approaches the essence of ambiguity from the internal evidence of language itself with this statement: "This

underlying enigma (about the problems of motives) will manifest itself in inevitable ambiguities and inconsistencies about
the terms for motives. Accordingly what we want is not terms
that avoid ambiguity, but terms that clearly reveal the strategic
spots at which ambiguities necessarily arise."[2]

Lewis Thomas arrives at the same point from the evidence of
cybernetics in biology. He states that the single-stage transactions and single-purpose functions in cells and insects are not
systems that allow for deviating:

> Perhaps it is in this respect that language differs most sharply
> from other biologic systems for communication. Ambiguity
> seems to be an essential, indispensable element for the trans-
> fer of information from one place to another by words, where
> matters of real importance are concerned. It is often necessary
> for meaning to come through, that there be an almost vague
> sense of strangeness and askewness. . . . Only the human
> mind is designed to drift away in the presence of locked-on
> information, straying from each point in a hunt for a better,
> different point. If it were not for the capacity of ambiguity . . .
> we would have no way of recognizing the layers of counter-
> point in meaning.[3]

Third, the computer technology of data storage and retrieval
(to be considered differently from the computer in calculation)
has magnified the evidence of our poor use of language in everyday medicine. The fault was always there. Technology has made
it intolerably evident, but did not create it or correct it. There
has been an explosion in communicative artifacts, as well as in
vocabulary. Words have not become fewer, they have become
more. An uncontrolled tide of verbiage (the worse for its perpetual, instant retrievability) presently overwhelms our thinking and understanding. A verbal redundancy has brought an inessential ambiguity and a corrupting inexactitude, by which
crudities may receive three titles of approbation while the varied
subtleties in a situation go unnamed.

Burgess Gordon, from the AMA Current Medical Technology
study of medical records, finds that 29,000 different names are
used for the designation of 3,200 to 3,800 specific diseases and
170,000 adjectives, descriptors or modifiers are employed when

20,000 to 22,000 would suffice. He calls the progressive increase in redundancy a "vocabulary in explosion."

The case of the elderly shows that this redundancy may denote a poverty of understanding and description. There is a surface stereotyping by a shuffling of alternates rather than an exploration of subtle, distinct phenomena from a vocabulary and concepts of adequacy and precision. The error is disguised by a loose, noncriterial use of scientific terms. For example, odd behavior in a person eighty-five years old may be called senility, cerebral arteriosclerosis, or chronic brain syndrome. Cardiomegaly or nondescript EKG ST—T changes in the same person will be called "ASHD."[4]

The computer-based data bank has not corrected the situation but it has most usefully intensified our sense of urgency that something has to be done. It is the translation of this sense into the active voice—"We will have to do something about ourselves"—where the block occurs, but the momentum of our machinery may leave us no choice unless we wish to drown!

There is misunderstanding concerning the use of measurement and mathematics in medical care of the human being. Neither measurement nor mathematics have diminished man's humanity whether as patient or as physician, or as to the tie of language between them. Epidemiology is only as strong as the verbal specifics. Statistical controlled trials of treatment depend on exquisite description of the human variables. It could also be said that in individual patient care, measurement is the highest form of respect in our observational practice. Prior assumptions are put on the altar for vindication or for burning.

In an introduction to examining range of motion and muscle strength for first-year medical students, I make an additional point that the need for measurement, especially in clinical trials, drives us to pay more particular attention to people. There is nothing impersonalizing about clinical quantification. It is the sloppy approximation or "impression" that does the individuality of the patient less than justice.

Inconsistent or idiosyncratic clinical techniques and records are therefore not concessions to a patient's uniqueness, but reflect an unprofessional self-indulgence, for they substantially deprive our patients from contributing to, and benefiting from, the common pool or reference, and deprive us from sharing fully or accurately the experience of others.

Last of all, cybernetics, the science of communication and organization, reveals deficiencies in the construct of our means, that only reconceptualization of the ends can hope to correct. Stafford Beer in *Platform for Change*,[5] expands the need for a mediating "metalanguage," one that will define human needs and goals operationally as well as humanly, thus harnessing the wasted resources of our technology for "edification" (to use the old biblical word) and not for mere profit and secondary ends. Here language turns back upon the metric and calls it to account. "Measure eudemony not money," says Beer, when you want to gauge medical care. Money, he argues, is an inferior metric, a containment, a restriction, a measure of the system of procurement only. "Measure what you really want to do and obtain in well-being." Is well-being (eudemony) measurable? We must define it first, explicate it, particularize it. Or is it only the "hard" inferior systems that are so definable? If so they will trap us as if they were themselves the ultimate end.

If medical care is concerned ultimately with well-being, its language and measurements will have to be stretched a lot yet. Certainly they cannot afford to part ways. Exactitude cannot be abandoned, even if to maintain it slows the pace. Consistency must address a constant flux of biologic activity, which it must never permanently freeze for the sake of convenience. Striving always for further resolution of inessential ambiguity, language and measurement have to accept Heisenberg's uncertainty principle as operative in human biology as in particle physics. Confident and secure in themselves so as to provide practical effect in the everyday world of sickness and health, they should also describe its diversity and unexpectedness.

Language and measurement are somewhat in tension and their professional users need to live with these tensions fruitfully, not seeking relief by abandoning one end or the other, so that practical utility is lost because the measurement of certainty is never judged complete, or so that exploration is denied because the security of existing categories is threatened. In truth, the real tensions are probably not between language and mea-

surement. That could be a contrived rivalry to spare the complacent, or the lazy, or the fearful the effort of their proper double
use in medicine.

To a large extent, the dialogists' understanding of Ian Lawson's paper was supplemented by his statements at the first meeting about his record-keeping system at the Hebrew Home for the
Aged and in his previously published essay, "A Taxonomy of
Geriatric Care."

We recognized his consistent concern that medical language
be convenient and yet also a reasonably accurate representation
of the complexities flesh is heir to. Ian felt that the best medical
records use some combination of the accuracy "provided by numbers (lab results, algorithmic decision trees, etc.) and the quality
provided by those who revere language." Just what that quality
was made for a little discussion among the dialogists. At one
point, Ian spoke of "poetic license," which upset Elizabeth until
she was satisfied that he also acknowledged something very like
"scientific license." Denise, too, objected to Ian's implication
that "those who revere language"—poets, for instance—might
provide some quality other than accuracy. She quoted Wallace
Stevens to the effect that "to be at the end of fact is not to be at
the beginning of poetry, but at the end of both."

Clearly, we were back at our polarities. Once again certain
members of the group made attempts to dispense with them, but
Ian added this sobering statement: "I speak of polarities as an
institutional fact." He assured us that built into the health care
institution is a tension between subjective and objective reporting, between imagination as part of assessing a patient's condition and measurement as part of pinpointing it precisely. Elizabeth was adamant in her response that Sloth, one of the deadly sins, was simply the inability to live with tension; whereas
Nancy suggested that we grab at numbers because we are terri-
fied of the unknown.

For her part, Denise wondered if the way doctors use language
and the way poets use it have anything in common at all and
suggested that the best thing the two groups could do for each
other was to demonstrate the differences. Perhaps therein lay

the dialogue. Sometime in the middle of our afternoon meeting, she reached for some paper and wrote this draft of a poem, entitled "Artist to Intellectual (Poet to Explainer)":[6]

I

"Don't want to measure, want to be
the worm slithering wholebodied
over the mud and grit of what
may be a mile,
may be forever—pausing
under the weeds to taste
eternity, burrowing
down not along,
rolling myself
up at a touch, outstretching
to undulate in abandon to exquisite rain,
returning, if so I desire, without
reaching that goal the measurers
think we must head for. Where is
my head? Am I not
worm all over? My own
orient!"

II

"Do I prophesy? It is
for now, for no future.
Do I envision? I envision
what every seed
knows, what shadow
speaks unheard
and will not repeat
My energy
has not direction,
tames no chaos,
creates, consumes, creates
unceasing its own
wildfires that none
shall measure."

III

"The lovely obvious! The feet
supporting the body's tree and its crown
of leafy flames, of fiery
knowledge, roaming
into the eyes,
that are lakes, wells, open
skies! The lovely
evident, revealing
everything, more mysterious
than any
clueless inscription scraped in stone.
The ever present, constantly vanishing,
carnal enigma!"

Reactions to this poem were fascinating. Most of us tried to behave calmly, but everyone seemed delighted that as a group we had somehow aided in the creation of a poem in our midst. Dick—the doctor, the celebrant—was the first to respond. His comment was one he might have hoped for from the group when he had read his story to us at Meeting Two: "I don't think *you*, Denise, should measure or be measured. It would never enhance; it could only detract from what is already there." Nancy murmured: "Her 'measure' and our 'measure' are different 'measures,'" but no one asked her to explain just what she meant, or even with whom she was aligning herself by saying "our." Presumably she meant the doctors versus Denise. But other groups were subtly forming, and Nancy could have been alluding to them.

For instance, Denise addressed her poem to intellectuals and explainers, not to doctors specifically. And Elizabeth, for one, may have understood "intellectuals" and "explainers" to mean "academics," who, she said—present company excepted—often made her despair. When Denise added as an afterthought to her poem, "I want to do rather than to know," she might have inadvertently underscored this new grouping into stereotypical artists, on the one side, and stereotypical academics, on the other.

79

But before the artists in the group (whether writers or not) could be ranged for dialogue with the explainers (whether teachers or not), the group came together in the evening to consider Elizabeth's paper on magic, and was once again realigned for a new conversation. Gene Moss, exhausted, excused himself and went to bed early, saying, "I'll see where you are in the morning." When he rejoined us, we were not quite in the same place.

PRELIMINARY REFLECTIONS ON MAGIC AND MEDICINE
Elizabeth Sewell

I want to ask you if you can agree to at least some of the following: all of us, here in this place and everywhere in all places of Western education—raised and permeated by a metaphysic more powerful because we are quite unaware of it—would deny that we were steeped in any metaphysic (or final unquestioned view of "reality") at all. From this metaphysic emerges a method, from which all our serious study goes on. Although all-powerful, it is also unrecognized.

If we are to think about magic, images and powers, imagination, we are going to have to shift from the unquestioned metaphysic and the unexamined method. Before we begin, three suggestions might help in the transition: "The nature of the visionary Imagination is very little known!"

"Imagination is a very new faculty."

"One might think of the Chinese and Western traditions travelling substantially the same path towards the science of today. But on the other hand—they might have followed, and be following, rather separate paths, the true merging of which lies well in the future."

Any attempt to shift method cannot be accomplished through critical expository prose addressed to the isolated reason. For this reason,I have included a poem and the beginning of a narrative here, not as objects of scrutiny but as exercises in transformation. The first I wrote years ago, the second records thoughts for something not yet embarked upon.

Image Imagination!
  Try if you can
Uncover weedgrown pathways,
  Unreason's plan,
Some recondite relation
  Of god and man.

          Image Imagination?
            Perhaps one should;
          But will you, from a planet,
            A darkening wood,
          Perceive the integration
            Of bad and good?

Image Imagination!
  You must divine
Man-Woman star-encrusted,
  Love's androgyne,
Clouds of intoxication
  In skies of wine.

          Image Imagination?
            How can one so?
          On these untravelled summits
            Fierce sun and snow
          Shrivel black lips' narration
            Of what they know.

Image Imagination!
  Bodies must turn
To force of naked water
  Through intellectual fern
In whose gesticulation
  Cold rainbows burn.

          Image Imagination—
            Then bind my wrists
          And, bound, with pain and blindness
            For catalysts,
          I hymn the consummation
            Of all that exists.

We were lost. How this had happened, and so suddenly, was not easy to understand. It was still early afternoon, our customary walk had taken us down to the Spreadeagle Falls as it often did, the waters frothing and clamoring over their seventy feet of rounded boulders. For all its energy this was somehow a snubby or chubby cataract, good for children, presenting no terror except perhaps the Himalayan cold of the stream's temperature. We had turned to walk back the quarter of a mile to the one-floor wood bungalow in the English compound where home was this summer; our *ayah* had murmured something about going for a little visit—up this path—to see "a cousin" of hers.

"Rampieri, how is it that you have a cousin who lives here?"

But we, trained to obey her grumpy patience, had turned with her. Now her white-swathed form seems also to have vanished among the dark trees, the lovely mountain pines, their needles brown and scented all around. The path is perceptible, and that's something. Only when paths start to disappear does panic begin. Already though, as the path extends its noncommittal self, comes a rather alarming tiredness. Afternoon walks are not usually this long, and there will be home yet to find and to walk to. Meanwhile, follow the path. It seems to be leading to an edge, of sorts, out from under the canopy, hanging low, of curving coniferous boughs.

I am holding to the path myself. I mean to keep my own rather strong legs and small feet firmly in it, trusting no one not to lose me further. The other two range out a little in the open wood, one on either hand. Leftwards from me is the little one. She has picked up something as she walks—a stone? minute speckled shard of bird's egg? a wad of red-tufted moss? —and is examining it in her cupped hands as she walks, slipping occasionally on the slippery needle-floor, and from time to time jerking her chin up to see she does not walk into one tree or another, and each time she does it, gleams from her long blonde hair signal to me as I march steadily along the path. The glimpses of that bodily brightness help me to keep her in view. That is more difficult with the one on my right. That is my other sister—oh, the young one's name is Minka. This on the right is Ferle and she is hard to keep track of because she is dressed in dark grey, wound round her in her queer fashion, and besides she is rather bent and slow.

Nevertheless she looks, curiously, as if she is moving forward by dint of nose and ears (both sharp) almost smelling or listening her way, so that she, by far the eldest of the sisters, is using her senses more acutely than we, the other two, I in my wariness, Minka in her curiosity. Ferle is fifty years older than I am, here in the middle, and I am that much older than our sharp and skipping six-year-old.

We are coming towards light, afternoon sun diffusing; to a clearing, I suppose. Minka reaches it first, running up a little bank and running down, catapulting into the circle of the glade, and as I emerge, pushing apart the rather thorny underbrush which is already the glade's life, not the forest's, I see Ferle hover out and then glide forward in her turn, a little farther down. At least if the three of us are lost we are all still together.

The clearing, if that is what it is, turns out, even on first glance, to be enormous, so wide the light changes as one looks across it, the far darkness of the tree boundary taking on a tinge of purple. There are people here! (Why should there not be?) They are certainly not Rampieri's cousins. Nor ours.

Running up to me now Minka, a little frightened. She takes me by the elbow.

"Are they—are they peacocks?"

I see why she asks. They do move slowly, glide trailingly their long robes, or plumage, spread behind them over the carpeted arena of earth, in pairs or small groups, a noble carriage of breast and head, and the head might almost carry, at this distance, the delicate crown of royalty borne by those great birds (who would be at home here).

"No, Minka. I see what you mean, though. What extraordinary colors"—indigo, purples, jade-green, a dark flame, saffron, a kind of blood-crimson—"Whoever are they?"

"Stars in the crystalline heaven." Ferle's voice, only just audible.

Turning towards her, I took fright myself for a moment. There were stars visible in the afternoon sky. I took in fifteen or twenty at a glance, faint but unquestionably present. Supernovae— impossible.

"Their names," Ferle went on, "Alhazen, Algazel, Alcor, Altair, Alpharetz, Averroes, Algol, Avicenna, Aldebaran, Alphard,

Alkindi, Albiruni, Alfarabi, Avenzoar." Chanted quietly, the words like a dumb music spun threads between the airy and brilliant forms sprinkled across both fields. "Star-led wizards," Ferle said. She has countless scraps of poetry in her mind.

So Ferle knows the names, of some at least; and some, though not many, of the circling figures, are women. Minka is chastened by a certain appropriate fear. We can perhaps approach a little closer.

At present the space and procession seem to center around one in the midst who sits on a rock there, one of the many bare old outcrops on this plain. Coming closer, one notices a small spring at the foot of the rock. One reads these signs. I glance at Minka to see she is going to behave. I need not worry: she will behave best of all of us.

Full white hair and beard, dark eyes that follow the wandering groups circling, talking. A long slim wooden rod rests against the rock beside him. One hand plays gently with a chain hanging from his waist, from which dangles something that rattles, chink chink, rhythmically against the rock. Almost in spite of myself I start counting those beats, one, two, three, four—I cannot see what the metallic thing is. Keys? Writing implements? He is dressed in full silk, blackish or gold as the light takes it, and sown all over it are small gold plates, about the size of the palm of a child's hand.

"Peacock!" Minka whispers urgently to me again. She has noticed, first of any of us, that on each of the thin gold discs is engraved an eye. Some are open, some closed.

"Argus!" is my response, whispered to her.

Ferle says, "Pythagoras."

He does not look up at any of the names. If so, this one admitted women from the beginning. And enjoined, upon all who were his, years of silence, did he not? I sit down, to wait.

What happens, gradually, is twofold. The noble figure moves, takes the rod, traces on the bare earth near his own bare feet, or retraces for it seemed as if it were there before, the triple triangle, the star pentagon. Ferle sets her hands together, lifts them to her forehead and bows lower from where she is crouched.

"The greeting," she murmurs, to Minka and myself. "Health." Then after a pause, "Also, the universe."

But meanwhile a second thing is happening. If you are silent, you hear. If you are silent, you listen. A sensation of something in the air, dropping down from above or netted by the wandering mazes of those others, it feels like a current of warmer or cooler air on the skin, setting it tingling, its own sensation the only perceived reality. I may be the one who knows least of it, so attend to the others, to Minka who might be hearing a flute playing somewhere far over towards the dark woods, to Ferle who is curling up one corner of her mouth, in delight or concentration upon some faint but cosmic harmony just and only just apprehended.

I sit silent, waiting, listening.

The tradition I am trying to reach back to could be said to be the tradition of all traditional societies, of which ours is not one. This "magic" (a convenient name for me to use) is the high magic, *magia*, of the Renaissance; the magic of, among others, men such as Ficino, Bruno or Paracelsus. It is not black magic, *goetia*. It is not charlatanry, just as we shall assume that medicine is not quackery. I am going to set out a list of some whom I know I need to learn about, and learn principally from, this high magic. I know already a good deal about two or three of them, a little about a few more, almost nothing about many—this just to say how much of a beginner I am.

The list is not strictly chronological, especially in the middle. Zoroaster, Orpheus, Hermes Trismegistus (and behind him, Thoth), Pythagoras, Empedocles, Plato, Iamblichus, Pseudo-Dionysius, Proclus, Porphyry, Plotinus, then the great Arabs whom I have already named (some at least, in these pages, though one should add Gebir for alchemy)—Gemisthus Pletho, Ficino, Pico della Mirandola, Agrippa, Paracelsus, Giordano Bruno, Campanella, John Dee, Shakespeare, Spenser, Bacon, Milton, possibly the Cambridge Platonists, Newton, Leibnitz, Vico, Blake, Coleridge, Thomas Taylor, Shelley, Yeats. I think Novalis and Goethe both belong here somewhere, as I am sure do Descartes of the dreams and the relationships with the Rosicrucians, and Mersenne with his music, going back to the Academies of the century preceding his, in Italy and in Paris.

Many of the works of these men are appallingly difficult to

find. Many are untranslated, let alone published here. We call the line "occult." What has hidden it? I think not the secretive or even noisome nature of its tenets, viewed from another perspective (though one thinks of how Gnostic texts appear to have been deliberately suppressed by, for instance, Christian authorities; how Pletho's masterwork was burned by a Byzantine church official—and so on). My dear and honored mediators into much of this, and I want to mention them here, are Frances Yates ("The modern world is dying for lack of magic") and Kathleen Raine in her glorious work on Blake and, more succinctly, in her prefaces to *Blake and Tradition* and *Thomas Taylor the Platonist* (with George Mills Harper). This, the Hermetic Neoplatonic, magical tradition is "occult" also because it ran counter to the prevailing religion the West early adopted, to Aristotelian ways of thought and Erasmian humanism, and counter to the metaphysic we adopted later when our religion collapsed.

This magical method sees the universe as network upon network, all open to each other, each resonating to other in a series of ordered systems, the whole a vast harmony, so that the two pervasive images for this cosmos are mathematics (for the network) and music (for the harmony and correspondence). Each element in the cosmos is alive—

> Of World and Mind
> Poet by poet said,
> "No thing is only dead,
> And nothing unrelated"

—according to its own due form. I think also that each is endowed with certain powers (magic is clearly operative, seeking in man to recognize powers we have by nature but have forgotten or have not yet divined), so that everything is reciprocally capable of exercising power upon (and is subject to that of) other objects and beings. The imagination in the human creature is the center of these powers. Since the method is reticular and not linear, this fact affects how cause and effect, and the nature of time, are seen. It tends to rule out chance and accident, viewing the latter, in Schopenhauer's words, as "Necessity that has come a longer way round." Determinism can be a problem for this

86

kind of thought, which is why men like Pico attacked dogmatic astrology. The network means that everything in the universe is, so to speak, porous:

> The rule, we find,
> Is to be permeable; marbles stain,
> Light filters through packed crystals;
>   someone's pain
> Threads our interstices . . .
> Stars sift across our system twice a day . . .

There is no line between inner and outer: "Though it appears without, it is within"; "In every bosom a universe expands as if with wings." All things are at once themselves, alive, and (if they are not pure spirit) matter and spirit. Since all are connected by varying relationships, the imagination is at its most discerning when it works by means of analogies, synthesis, symbols, images themselves.

Medicine? And how on earth does that great activity tie up, as our modern minds might ask slightly aghast, with all this? I don't yet clearly know, and don't want to make pronouncements about medicine at all, which is not my faculty as poetry is. I want to ask myself questions, though, in the light of what our group is asking about. How do we, and how might we, imagine ourselves into health (and no doubt into sickness, but that is vastly less important here)? What do we make of the long tradition which has held that there is a central relationship between medicine and all the elements of this tradition—the magus / physician comes to mind, historically and imaginatively to be attended to; Pythagoras was one such; so was Empedocles; what went on at places like Cos and Epidauros—theatre and dreams and natural beauty and ritual as an inherent part of effecting a change, perhaps, in the patient's imagination? Did you know (I didn't till very recently) that most of the great Arab sages were physicians, Avicenna and Averroes in chief, giving its double sense to *hakim*, the physician and philosopher-magus-alchemist —or know that Maimonides, besides being the great philosopher he was, served also as physician to Saladin's vizier? How about Dr. Faustus, in Marlowe and Goethe, where legendary and numerous cures are part of the character makeup? And Prospero who "heals" the brains, "boiled in their skulls," of erring men on his island? And the woman physician in *All's Well that Ends Well*? And the other late Shakespearian plays might have suggestions, too.

What if, in a musicalized universe, the function of medicine as of education with which it is closely connected, were the elimination of discords, the restoration of inner and outer harmony— "O may we soon again renew that song / And keep in tune with Heaven"—in a world where doctor and patient saw themselves and each other as (as Owen Barfield suggests) not islands, but something more like embryos within nature, the permeability image again? How would it affect their mutual work? How much time does medicine now spend trying to undo the ill effects of our present image of ourselves and our nature, individual and communal, which is inherent in presentday society? Could it be better occupied?

Much of what I have said seems to relate to "preventive medicine." I think we might also want to ask about those matters we tend to avoid: the proliferation of healing "cults" today; drugs; the passivity or helplessness the patient feels the moment after being admitted to hospital in which the physician-patient relationship is not cooperative; and the attitude towards death.

DICK SELZER   I want to know more about Ferle and Minka. Who are they and which parts of your imagination do they represent? They seem to be extraordinary, sensitive, perceptive little machines and to know something the rest of us don't know.

ELIZABETH SEWELL   I think the answer to that, Dick, is that you will have to think of who yours are.

DICK SELZER   Why does Ferle say "Pythagoras"?

ELIZABETH SEWELL   She knows who it is. There is a legend that Pythagoras visited India. It is undoubtedly Pythagoras who is the sage at the center.

NANCY ANDREASEN   Why doesn't he respond when she recognizes him?

ELIZABETH SEWELL   Because I don't know what he says: I'll have to wait and hear. I've done this sort of thing before. When you're talking to Bacon or Coleridge, you've got bags of stuff that they say. But with Pythagoras I'll have to wait and see.

DENISE LEVERTOV   Was this a dream?

ELIZABETH SEWELL   No, it was not a dream. It just appeared.

DICK SELZER   You and your sisters—what are you after? What are you seeking? I take this to be an exploration into terra incognita. I feel myself being seduced by your language. You're hinting to us all along. And yet you don't come right out and say what it is you're thinking. I suppose it's magic that's the way into this witchy business.

ELIZABETH SEWELL   It's the high tradition of magic. And that's why Pythagoras and the Arabic sages and the stars are there. It is also to some extent scientific. The astronomy of the tradition is there, and if we go on talking long enough, we'll come to medicine and alchemy, and I don't know what else we'll come to.

IAN LAWSON   Is your view of high magic one of a replacement for the metaphysic which you see as absent (and I agree is absent) from our present thinking? And how is it different from the orthodox hierarchies of religion?

ELIZABETH SEWELL   High magic is a way of thinking about a different metaphysic. Its theology is closer to the cabalistic in that there is the unknown and unknowable first principle, imaged as the sun, but it is not the visible sun. It is some great center and is also within every man.

   I wrote this paper to tell you what I know, but there is a great deal I don't know. This is my next five or ten years' work. And I think the center of the work will be Giordano Bruno. I think he is going to be my master for the next five or ten years.

DICK SELZER   Who was Giordano Bruno?

ELIZABETH SEWELL   He was a renegade Dominican born about

1550, became interested in magical memory, a strong tradition in the Dominican order. Then he began to travel. In Paris he became involved in court circles. Fascinated with the worlds of myth and magic, Bruno's first books became treatises on myth and memory. Travelling to England, he joined the circle of Philip Sidney. There he developed a great cult of Queen Elizabeth, and was right in the midst of that strange court magic prevalent in the masqes. These experiences helped him to write perhaps his three greatest books. Once in Germany, Bruno pursued magic as a power of the human mind, as the great hermetic tradition, and memory as a part of that tradition. He drew illustrations for his own books. In all his work, Bruno was trying to find, or get back to, an old religion. In fact, he might have been burned at the stake for trying to start a new religion.

DENISE LEVERTOV What was the role of memory in what he thought?

ELIZABETH SEWELL One of the earliest of the hermetic texts speaks about powers which the ancient Egyptian priests could summon from above. These powers, actually starry influences, were transformed into images. Now this story can be taken simply as idolatry or as an attempt to explain what actually happens in the mind and the magic and power of images working therein. The result is some statement about imagination and memory, which of course works by images. Behind this statement lie the great arts of memory as described by Quintilian, I think. Later there developed fantastic systems for giving memory enormous powers, so as to stimulate the imagination. With these powers come ones of prophecy, and the business of storing and organizing images within the mind. Bruno's religion had four principles: magic, art, mathematics with a magical turn, and love. It was developed partly in reaction against the appalling excesses of the wars of religion, the obscenity and cruelty then in progress. In reading Newton's alchemical studies this past summer, I noticed that this tradition runs as a steady thread through all the great scientists.

JIM COWAN   But even now there are still books being written to show that witchcraft, alchemy, astrology, etc., have no basis in scientific validity of any sort. I'm suspicious of books in which older scientific traditions are rejected as charlatanry, or when writers fail to see the intellectual and spiritual elements in the entire hermetic tradition.

ELIZABETH SEWELL   This rejection can only occur if you keep the two sorts of reality separate. The alchemists' attempt to make gold and the attempt, as it were, to purify one's spirit seem to us two separate things, but in fact they're not, and that's why we have to put them back together.

AL VASTYAN   Is there any accessibility to the truth of the high tradition except through a deep commitment to one propounding that truth in a very personal way? I am impressed by your saying in effect that you are going to indenture yourself to Giordano Bruno as a master.

ELIZABETH SEWELL   In the first place, "truth" gives me trouble. I'm not sure that's the right word. I've served as apprentice to Coleridge as master for ten years, and I've been serving a brief apprenticeship to Blake.

DENISE LEVERTOV   But why do you have to look for a master?

ELIZABETH SEWELL   It presents itself in that light to me. My imagination sees itself as somehow belonging in that line. When you apprentice yourself to people you naturally talk to them a great deal. The last book I wrote—one I can't get published—is a record of conversations I've had with Coleridge. It's a statement, partly, about how such poets can be studied. I have a sense that poets can be studied. I have a sense that poets are not dead. I want to get rid of my sense of linear time.

DENISE LEVERTOV   In this book about Coleridge, how much do you have a sense of literal communion, and how much are you putting into his mouth?

ELIZABETH SEWELL   The work was reading Coleridge and taking notes. But I like to move into where my masters are—that's why I sent you this fable we're talking about now. The fiction was a great house in a landscape Coleridge describes.[7] He talks about a young friend, a student. They come to where the land falls away into deep water—it's a coastal landscape. Then he says to the young student, "Now, friend, you've walked this far with me just for exercise or conversation. It's time you found your way home, for this is where the great adventure starts. Here is neither boat nor raft, but out there waiting for us is a great ship. The ship is Philosophy, and it is to take us to the Fortunate Isles." You realize that Coleridge sees this whole life of the mind as a voyage of adventure, as Vico did, as perhaps Shakespeare does in *The Tempest*. And you realize that "The Rime of the Ancient Mariner" is some sort of extraordinary voyage of understanding about how Coleridge thought. The house is a mind. You can live in Coleridge's mind if you want to. In a way it's a vision of how I study people—you may love your master, but there is no reason whatever why your master should love you. How the Pythagoras thing is going to work out, I don't know, but it's obviously a further venture of the same kind.

DICK SELZER   I'm having trouble with all of this. I think it's dangerous, that's one word for it. I think it's insane, that's another word. Elizabeth, you have a scholarly interest in this long tradition. But there is something else going on. And my trouble here tonight comes from trying to see where the academic, scholarly pursuit ends, and the real magic begins.

ELIZABETH SEWELL   I don't think that there is a line. That's why I set the story into the paper I sent all of you, so as not to send you just a scholarly piece. I have to walk into whatever I do. Imaginative fusion is part of my scholarly method. Insanity is part of my method.

NANCY ANDREASEN   I wish you all wouldn't use that term so loosely!

JO TRAUTMANN   "Madness" isn't a bad word to use here, because it has a long tradition of moonlight and inspiration.

DICK SELZER Am I the only one who is recoiling a bit from what Elizabeth is saying? What about you, Denise?

DENISE LEVERTOV I'm not recoiling from it exactly. It seems that there are people whom I know, like and respect, who are extremely knowledgeable—much more scholarly than I am—who make me suppose that their way of operating as creative human beings is to live out their metaphors to a point in which they are unable to answer such questions as, "where does scholarship end and faith begin?" Though I've written poetry all my life, and know myself to be a good poet and an imaginative person—I don't have that need to live this kind of metaphor. I'm much more ordinary. So I can only look on with a certain amount of awe, but also with a certain amount of indifference!

NANCY ANDREASEN I steeped myself in that tradition for a number of years, not as much as Elizabeth has or will, but when she speaks, I remember the wonder and the excitement.

JO TRAUTMANN Did you also flee this tradition when you left literature for psychiatry?

NANCY ANDREASEN It fled me.

IAN LAWSON Now this business of telling the future: it's a cherished medical craft, based upon sensory evidence. As I hear it, prognostication in the magical sense is based upon secret evidence which seems attainable only by entrusting oneself without knowing the ethical price. This seems to be one big difference between medicine and magic.

ELIZABETH SEWELL One is always committing oneself to the unknown.

NANCY ANDREASEN One can't always give informed consent.

30 January 1976
The issues raised by Ian's and Elizabeth's papers and Denise's poem were considered in a variety of ways at the morning session. For instance, Jim Cowan rose at dawn to write us the following memorandum, in which he deals not only with the pre-

vious day's discussion but also with his reactions to the first two meetings.

THE APOLLONIAN AND THE DIONYSIAN

James C. Cowan

In his first book, *The Birth of Tragedy* (published in 1872), Friedrich Nietzsche speaks of two opposing aesthetic worlds which he named for two Greek divinities of art: the Apollonian and the Dionysian. These choices were made so as to facilitate identification of two opposite kinds of art—the first, epical and pictorial and the second, musical and balletic—which developed in classical Greece and which evolved side by side. Ultimately in the genius of the Hellenic mind, they were fused in an art equally Apollonian and Dionysian: Attic Tragedy. Nietzsche uses the word "dream" (in its pre-Freudian sense as a formal, pictorial given) to denote the Apollonian world; and the word "intoxication" (in the sense of rapture) to denote the Dionysian world.

Drawing on recent research I did on D. H. Lawrence's dualism in terms of these two opposing worlds (which I think must be reconciled in all great art), I'd like to make the following points: (1) The Apollonian view assumes a linear development that is rational and logical, built upon *analysis* and depending on the conscious mind, with an objective, knowable truth as a reachable end point; (2) the Dionysian view assumes a cyclic development that is intuitive and imaginative, built upon creative *synthesis* and depending on unconscious modes of experience, with a subjective, even a revealed, truth that can never be expressed in abstract or conceptual language but only embodied in the concrete images that Susanne K. Langer calls "presentational symbols."

One may live in what is perceived as a world of Apollonian rationality, using the language of science and measurement, of truths validated in the laboratory; or, if you will, a world of grammar, literary scholarship, and methods of criticism. But what if experience should be fractured by an exception? What if the logical stairway with which we were so familiar led not here, as we had learned to expect, but there? Then we are confronted with an exception, a Dionysian experience of something—whether it be god, ghost, or void—that does not fit our neat schema of experience, and the result is a spontaneous response of awe or reverence or wonder.

We are all of us, I believe, programmed by our education and our society to disbelieve that kind of experience, despite the fact that we pay lip service to it in church and have evidence of it in the lives of poets, saints, mystics, and madmen. Do you know D. H. Lawrence's poem "Snake"? The golden snake, "crowned king in the underworld," enters the speaker's consciousness one hot Sicilian day by coming up for a drink. Although awed by the beauty of this Dionysian emissary, the speaker has to respond to what he calls "the voices of my education" and throws a stick at the snake, which retreats hastily into a fissure in the earth, leaving the speaker aware of his own pettiness. I think that as children all of us used to have such experiences of wonder—for example, in reading Grimm's fairy tales.

Dionysian perceptions are very easily lost, and there is no truth of any kind that cannot be turned into a lie—that is, made unfaithful to experience when it is condensed and packaged in *Reader's Digest* format. Nietzsche cites the wonderful statement of universal brotherhood in the "Ode to Joy" section of Beethoven's *Ninth Symphony* as an example of Dionysian rapture celebrating the reconciliation of Nature with her lost son, man. Unfortunately, such a statement can be reduced to the *Ladies' Home Journal* concept of "togetherness" because of its commercial usefulness. Even the God who spoke with St. Teresa and the Blessed Mother who appeared to St. Bernadette can be packaged and sold in a form acceptable to everyone and made to serve the ends of a commercial and materialistic secular order.

We live in a kind of organized unbelief that masquerades as belief. The flag stands at the center of our churches, in a place equal to that of the Cross, and sometimes even supersedes it as a sign of what we really worship, free enterprise and all that it implies for our way of thinking. Where the Church speaks of a communion of saints and Nietzsche speaks of a rapturous brotherhood, we now speak, in the cant phrases of the moment, of "the business community," "the academic community," "the medical community," and even "the intelligence community."

I am trying to identify these two opposing worlds of art and experience because I think that understanding them is important for our whole dialogue to date. Their opposed realities lie at the heart of the story Dick Selzer read at our second meeting, and in Bill Ober's response to it. Moved by the story and caught in the magical world Dick created wherein a Dionysian experience of communion between physician and patient signals the incursion of the unexpected and seemingly miraculous into the Apollonian world of hospital routine, I could not have *dis*believed the story. Whether literally true or not, I never questioned, because it was artistically true. Bill Ober, however, like an eighteenth-century rationalist or a modern pragmatist, was not caught in that world but in the world he knows so well, the pathologist's laboratory. "Where is the slide?" he asked. In a fury, I heard myself saying that at the heart of our differences in this dialogue group lay two world views which were totally opposed, not merely in the disagreement between Nancy Andreasen and me on the question of a dynamic psychological theory of human personality, nor in the disagreement between Dick Selzer and Bill Ober on the question of a miraculous cure, which Bill was compelled by "the voices of [his] education" to explain away ("if so, then it wasn't carcinoma, it was something else that looked like it"), but in two diametrically opposite and perhaps irreconcilable ways of viewing the whole world. The gulf between these opposing world views seemed so vast that I questioned whether it was even possible to bridge it.

But obviously I must think that it is in some measure possible to bridge the gulf, and so must you; otherwise we wouldn't be here. As soon as Ian Lawson spoke of illness as a positive condition of the whole patient and refused to reduce the patient to a set of governmentally approved diagnostic categories, he was making reconciliation between the two worlds possible in his own practice. The patient is still a person, not an abstraction, and Ian is still a person, not a functionary. As soon as Dick Selzer responded to the evidence of living experience on the part of a six-month fetus in an abortion and questioned his own liberal assumptions, which, though I don't like to think they are, can be equally as abstracting as, say, conservative assumptions, then reconciliation between the two worlds is possible.[8] I am using the word *reconciliation*—Coleridge's term is "reconciliation of opposites"—rather than Whitman's term "merge"—because, like D. H. Lawrence, I do not think that merger and fusion, or confusion, of the polarities is even desirable. Lawrence believed that truth, for both art and living, was to be found in the tension in balanced polarity between the two, and that it would be disastrous for either side to win a permanent victory over the other or for the two sides to lose their identity by merger and dissolution in each other. I think that when we make statements or enter into dialogue with each other, we need to make clear in what world we are speaking, and that as Elizabeth Sewell said in our second meeting, "None of us may say to the other, 'You are not real.'"

Denise Levertov's poem which she read to us yesterday opposes the world of measurement (Apollonian) and being (Dionysian). She feels, as Archibald MacLeish put it in "Ars Poetica," that "a poem should not mean / but be." It is as if measurement, analysis, and the rationalist approach to reality on which they are based presupposed a dead carcass of experience to dissect rather than a living being to experience in the cyclic Now. I understand her concern about that. Lawrence refers in *St. Mawr* to psychologists as, if I may paraphrase, pathologists of the psyche dissecting the soul. Yet Lawrence and Denise Levertov have their own kind of measurement. Some day critics will literally measure the prosody in Denise's new poem as they now do in all of Lawrence's poems. However internal and experiential their poetic rhythms, their awareness of line, meter, alliteration, assonance, rhyme, can be described objectively. They may literally *think* the symbols, experience all the poetic elements inwardly, and produce the poem as an imaginative Dionysian whole. The critic or scholar who approaches the poem from the opposite Apollonian point of view will analyze and discriminate, describe, and, it is to be hoped, make accessible to others the experience which the poet has embodied in presentational symbols. That the critic may do violence to the poem in the process, remains a possibility, as is the chance that rather than making the poem more accessible, he may simply interpose himself between the poet and his readers and students, standing as a kind of guard at the gate of their poetic experience.

Elizabeth Sewell talked with Coleridge. I awoke at five o'clock this morning thinking of that, for I have lived with D. H. Lawrence for many years now, learned from him and at times entered empathetically the world of his experience, but I have never talked with him. In the Apollonian world where I have lived most of my life, I am not attuned to alternative modes of knowing. The experience which Elizabeth describes as magic is not normally available to most of us, and when it occurs, "the voices of [our] education" cause doubts, and we throw sticks at it: "Where is your slide?" or "Do you mean this for real or for metaphor?" From a workaday perspective, the whole thing sounds a little crazy. No, there is no slide, though some people have another tradition, another discipline that can be evoked for such experiences as I have been nominating Dionysian. In western civilization the tradition has often been in effect a counter-religion to the established religion which served the purposes of the State or it would not have been tolerated. Examples were alchemy, white magic, and astrology. More recently in America, various offshoots of Eastern religions and meditative techniques have served this function. None of these are a direct part of my own experience, yet I accept them as, in some sense and for some people, real.

Metaphor is not an ornament; it is the essential truth of experience that the poet like Coleridge or Lawrence, Levertov or Sewell perceives and incarnates in concrete presentational image. After the fact, the rationalist may describe the experience, or the poem which sets it forth, in the conceptual language of discursive reasoning. But I question whether he can really get at the original experience in this way or even approximate it conceptually. I don't know. What I do know is that it is a mistake to take one kind of reality for the other, or the language of Dionysus for the language of Apollo. The psychiatrist may ask, "Do you experience these voices as coming from inside your own head or from the outside?" But this question presupposes the existence of the voices in the patient's reality. A healthy respect for the patient and his reality seems to me necessary if doctor and patient are to communicate at all, let alone do each other any good.

I certainly don't want to suggest that there is no such thing as mental illness or to say, like Thomas Szasz, that it is a myth. But what sort of hubris leads us to put every alternative kind of experience in a box labeled *madness*, and our own routine which we have found necessary to our world view in another box labeled *sanity*? In William Faulkner's *As I Lay Dying*, Cash Bundren comments:

> Sometimes I ain't so sho who's got ere a right to say when a man is crazy and when he ain't. Sometimes I think it ain't none of us pure crazy and ain't none of us pure sane till the balance of us talks him that-a-way. It's like it ain't so much what a fellow does, but it's the way the majority of folks is looking at him when he does it.[9]

Emily Dickinson wrote that she had tasted "a liquor never brewed." I am prepared to accept that statement. She tasted it whether I say so or not, and whether I even understand her taste or not. If I am a good critic and a reasonable man, I must turn to the evidence of her poetry as the embodiment of the truth of her experience. And possibly there is a judicious critical language that may help me in reconciling her experience and mine.

LETTER FROM WILLIAM B. OBER TO THE DIALOGISTS

. . . Re Jim's Apollo / Dionysus: It's an old dichotomy, a bit simplistic, and I think people take Nietzsche far too seriously. Thomas Mann's *Death in Venice* may have been a blue ribbon exhibit circa 1910, but half a century later it's pretty badly faded. I don't agree that I respond with "awe or reverence or wonder" when I'm confronted with a Dionysian experience. If it's agreeable, I respond like a pagan hedonist and ask for more. If it's not agreeable (or if I'm indifferent to it), I am rather casually dismissive. I suppose my problem is that I was raised in Boston in the 1920s and early 1930s and that much as I enjoy being a pagan hedonist as often as I can, that Puritan ethic still lingers here and there, and I'm an incomplete or failed pagan hedonist.

But I tried. A pathologist's trade makes him a voyeur, and it is the specific empirical sensation that counts most with me. Something to be seen, touched, felt, heard, or tasted (my sense of smell isn't much good). I tend to distrust transformations of sensory experience that get too far away from the initial stimulus (*The Diabelli Variations* may be top notch, but Beethoven does wander a bit far.) But Jim's piece is good and filled with provocative ideas. It is all very well and good for Emily Dickinson to say that she tasted a liquor never brewed, etc., but I would rather walk hand-in-hand with Thackeray through *Vanity Fair* than sail with Yeats to Byzantium. Either one is a good trip.

Recollections
Less Madness and More Art
The Doctor-Writer

30 April– 1 May 1976

Our fourth meeting began with remembrances of the third. Although we had responded to Elizabeth Sewell's paper on medicine and magic, we hadn't dealt directly with the issues Elizabeth brought up in her last paragraphs—those questions about the ways in which the old traditions she partly revived for us could be connected to medicine as practiced today. Nor did we respond much more directly when we met this time. But because the dialogue, however oblique, challenged medicine and literature in ways neither discipline is comfortable with, part of the discussion is reproduced here. Jim Cowan's application of the Apollonian-Dionysian distinction was also in our minds, and seemed related to Elizabeth's position or at least what others perceived to be her position.

Gene Moss brought two papers. The first, on madness, follows later and is in part a refocusing of the subject as discussed at Meeting Two. The second was an edited version of a presentation made in March 1975 at the University of Florida. This presentation was referred to in the Prologue as the occasion on which Gene suggested that the medical view of the patient is essentially, even inevitably, comic, but that from the patient's point of view, his or her situation is closer to the tragic. That had been an intriguing thought, teasingly brief as Gene had expressed it then. The edited paper expanded and changed the idea: "Tragedy focuses attention on the individual life, and thereby gives value to it. Comedy is more concerned with the processes of human life, wherein the individual is regularly *only* a part. The problem now revolves around the loss of the tragic structure from the experience of living and from the arts. In some measure, the future of health care will depend upon how modern society can provide intensity and meaning for its members—people who too often lead lives of irrelevance and indifference. I wonder how many patients come to the health care system with such a complaint. I wonder how many come longing for the meaning and intensity that only the tragic can provide."

Gene's second paper seemed to be in some of the dialogists' minds throughout the session and possibly accounted for the turn of the conversation.

The final subject considered at this meeting was the doctor as writer. The group had one new paper on the subject, Jo Trautmann's essay on Chekhov, which she intended as a reaction to several of the topics raised at previous meetings. Also distributed was her previously published essay on William Carlos Williams,[1] in which she talks about the nature of objectivity in medicine and art as practiced by this doctor-writer.

JO TRAUTMANN   Elizabeth's paper is not an analytical one, by any means, and neither do we in responding to it have to be restrictively analytical. I think we ought to relax into a discussion and just see where it takes us.

GENE MOSS   You know, to deal with these matters, with your paper, Elizabeth, requires an altogether different language for thinking about time and space. Immanuel Kant's two modes of perception just won't do.

ELIZABETH SEWELL   That's why my paper began as it did, saying to you, "Please try to become aware that you are boxed in here."

JIM COWAN   Let me speak for a minute on the two opposite sides of this question, for I see both of them clearly and equally. Since

Descartes, or whenever, we have more and more seen the universe itself as something to be dissected, to be analyzed, or to be measured in quantitative terms, and thus something to be manipulated. This is carried over from our attitude toward rocks and things like that to our attitude toward living organic nature, then is carried over to our children. They become things for us to manipulate and manage, and put through a particular sort of education. An ultimate result is behavioral modification in psychology, in which other people are seen as objects to be manipulated.

GENE MOSS   We see them as discrete too.

JIM COWAN   Yes, we don't see them as part of an organic universe, as part of a continuum with the universe, let alone as part of a continuum with us, as if we (doctor and patient, teacher and student) were, in Elizabeth's image, contained in a kind of embryonic sack together. And all that has its negative consequences.

On the other hand, if I may argue the other side for a moment, I think my life has been basically Apollonian. Any Ph.D's is, I think. In the same way that I think a doctor's is. Certainly a good surgeon, for instance, will relate to his patient's feelings and take the patient's being into account. In that sense, the patient might be a part of the surgeon. However, I suspect that when he goes into the O.R. and his responsibility is to do a certain surgical procedure, then his mind must pretty much screen out various other kinds of stimuli about the patient's family, person—and must concentrate on tying off blood vessels or whatever it is that he's doing. But really I don't think we can do without either one of these processes.

DICK SELZER   Do you think it is possible to think of the surgeon, when he is operating, as so fused, so permeable with his patient that when he operates on his patient he is in fact reconstructing himself? Does that idea mean anything to you?

JIM COWAN   Yes, I can accept that. But on the other hand I can see that a surgeon, in order to live, needs a certain kind of defense mechanism that allows him to screen off some things.

DICK SELZER   I am committed to the idea that a surgeon should avoid being a technocrat by all means, even if surgery has to be thought of in religious terms; that the doctor and the patient are pilgrims. Together they are in a search for the miracle of healing. For these reasons it has to be imbued with some higher purpose or flavor than technocracy.

JO TRAUTMANN   I wonder if this story has some relevance at this point: I once went with a former student—who had studied literature with me during medical school, and was now chief resident in surgery at the local city hospital—through one of her days, just because we had reached a point at which, if we were to continue working together, I had to know something of her world, as she knew of mine. In any case, one of the operations she performed that day was a mastectomy. And as Jane was cutting off the breast, I looked around the room and suddenly realized that everyone present was a woman: the patient; Jane, the surgeon; me, the observer. The medical student on that service happened to be a woman and the anesthesiologist, too. All the nurses were women. When the assistant was sewing up, Jane said, "Where is the breast?" and someone brought her a cup, a tin cup, which she overturned to slide the breast onto a table, and there all we women were huddled over this breast, and with my literary training—and no doubt my ritualistic imagination, you see—I said, "But this is Amazonian. All of us have just performed and witnessed an Amazonian operation. We have taken off our sister's breast," but then I stopped because I was getting looks that signaled, "This is what happens when a literature professor comes into the O.R., for God's sake." Some of them knew the ritual I was referring to; others didn't; but perhaps most of them thought I was being fanciful, whereas I felt that for myself at least the operation had been imagined into a new sphere. We women had come together with the patient and provided support for her and ourselves even as we cut off her breast.

DICK SELZER   It may be that the act of surgery was outrageous to the patient and to some extent to the surgeon, and it is possibly you, with your Amazonian perception, who may have had the third eye and seen through to the wisdom, the truth, of the situation. So I think it is as valid for you to make that perception as it is for the surgery team to be doing what they're doing. But we must not give their work, which is also my work, an excessive seriousness, an authority which it does not have.

NANCY ANDREASEN   Dick is seeing more of the humor in it, and you more of the horror.

JO TRAUTMANN   No. I didn't think it was horrible at all. As a matter of fact, I thought it was a more comprehensible act as a result of the Amazonian comparison. I thought it was: a) less disgusting; b) less terrifying; c) less the end of femininity; because the original Amazonian patient was not a victim at all, but had the operation to mark her as one of the women warriors, the archers.[2]

DICK SELZER   I can understand why some might have taken your statement as frivolous or distracting. I have performed the operation of mastectomy innumerable times, and each time something within me is shrieking. "Stop this, this is not natural; this is not normal; this serves no purpose." It is a terrible defilement of the flesh and, I think, the surgeon, in order to protect himself and stay sane, stay Apollonian, and not get into the madness, dare not confront this other aspect of it. And when someone violates that, as you did with your statement and your perception, and says something absolutely unutterable in that environment, you threaten these people in a profound way. They cannot hear it. They must denigrate you. They must laugh at you. They must departmentalize their thoughts.

JIM COWAN   That's what I was asking a while ago. Isn't this kind of departmentalizing necessary to function in that situation?

DICK SELZER   Well, we have this kind of Yankee horror of expressed compassion because—

JIM COWAN   You have a horror of what someone else will call "sentimental."

DICK SELZER   Yes, and because we're taught that it isn't func-

tional; that it is better to act silently; to take off a breast rather
than to dwell on the significance of it, or the literary significance of it.

NANCY ANDREASEN   There is a kind of tension behind this. I am
thinking of a doctor I know who committed suicide recently.
He was a highly sensitive person. What I want to know is if a
good deal of what doctors do isn't the kind of sensitivity we
are trying to encourage in this group. It is dangerous to think
and ponder and feel every time you cut a patient, to see when
you lose a patient that *you've* lost a life. To have this happen
again and again is the rock getting worn away. It's a human life
getting worn away.

DICK SELZER   I know that to be a fact. And yet woe betide the
patient whose surgeon forgets for one moment that there is a
living human being under those sheets with the same con-
flicts, wants, needs, and dreams as he himself has. Then the
act of surgery takes on a kind of violence to me, a sense of
cruelty, and a bloodiness that it ought not to have. Then one
runs the risk of embruing one's hands with gore.

NANCY ANDREASEN   But how far can a literature professor or a
writer—a humanist—ask a physician to go? That's really what
I'm asking. I'm seeing Elizabeth's paper as a plea or even a
demand for us to put ourselves in touch with this other perspective, these other forces, and I'm asking whether, if a physician does this, he can live with himself. Could you live with
the sense of disembodied organs surrounding you for the rest
of your life? Are you asking too much of people if they simultaneously have to do the acts and carry the imagination?

ELIZABETH SEWELL   I know that when we think of, say, physicians, and maybe others who come into daily contact with
immediate and appalling suffering, they provide a special case.
Yet Wordsworth says if you begin to take upon yourself the
anguish of the whole world, you are going to go crazy. You are
going to die. What we as humanists and physicians need is an
awareness of this fact without saying, "All right, I won't feel
any of this." But there's this dreadful balance—and it *is* dreadful—between the two, between Apollo and Dionysius, Nancy.

And I can't imagine why we feel that Apollo is safe! Apollo is one of the most dangerous gods. You can go equally mad with Apollo as you can with Dionysius. Nietzsche is so right on this point. He says we can't look at Dionysius. We must draw a veil across him, and Apollo is the veil. The whole issue revolved around tragedy. When I teach tragedy, I try to say to the students, "This is not something you just do for literary stuff; this is how one learns to manage the intolerable because by and large life is intolerable."

JO TRAUTMANN   I'm thinking through all this about Alvarez's book on suicide,[3] in which he states that certain artists take upon themselves some of these intolerable pains. They make it their business to pursue the pain on behalf of all of us till the end. And of course sometimes they don't come back. There have been studies describing doctors in the same light, essentially as scapegoats.[4] As a group, we have not wanted to see doctors as heroic figures, and we spent a session trying to dismiss sentimental views of suicide, but certainly many have seen both writers and doctors as similar bearers of our pain.

ELIZABETH SEWELL   The image of Jesus on the cross must have been marvelously helpful here because obviously he took it *all* on. We, neither the writer nor the physician, can take it all on—that would be hubris. And it's interesting that the Catholic tradition used the mother figure also, the Mater Dolorosa, you know, the figure with the seven swords in her heart? Catholics seem to have needed a feminine figure as well as the one on the cross. Jesus was not fully sufficient.

AL VASTYAN   Is the woman the only one who can image a continuity as well as a discontinuity? The male figure in the Christian religion is almost too nakedly alone.

ELIZABEH SEWELL   There are a few women in the tradition I'm interested in. One of the earliest is Circe, of course, and it's extraordinary what happens to her in the Renaissance. And I think it's Agrippa who speaks of the Sibyls as "magicianesses."

JO TRAUTMANN   Look, let's start this discussion again. Let's go back more directly to Elizabeth's paper and take some risks. I think we have to follow some of her suggestions out on some limbs and see what we come up with. She mentions preventive medicine, for one thing. And what a patient might be able to do to cooperate with the doctor, what sort of power a patient might have with respect to his or her own health. Does anyone have something to say on those topics, or any of the others? We won't have done our duty, in one way, or had as much fun, in another, if we don't take some chances that might lead to some silly statements, and perhaps to other things as well.

ELIZABETH SEWELL   Well, there is a navy doctor in San Francisco, who is a psychiatrist and working on imagination and health. And I hear there is a doctor in Texas [O. Carl Simonton] who is working on terminal cancer by means of the imagination. He is getting patients to think about their bodies, to think in terms that might be healing. It's been said that he has had some intriguing results.

DICK SELZER   There is an age-old and absolutely bona fide way for getting rid of warts, and that is to charm them. I have seen warts disappear on command. I know it's crazy, but, by God, under hypnosis warts go away if they're told to. I once had a wart on my toe, and I decided to charm it and every day I ordered it to go away. This is silly, but you asked for silly stories.

JO TRAUTMANN   What is the relationship between hypnosis and magic?

NANCY ANDREASEN   I've played around with hypnosis. To me, it is ultimately a form of charlatanry. I think that other people can make hypnosis work, but when I do it, I feel like a charlatan, so I've quit trying. But that's just me and says nothing about the overall issue of hypnosis. I think there's no question but that people can do a great deal by self-suggestion—I mean, they can suspend their ability to feel pain, if they can be so powerfully self-suggestive—which is what I think hypnosis really is. It involves another person helping someone to suggest himself into that state.

ELIZABETH SEWELL   "Hypnosis" is Greek, isn't it? It's "Sleep."

Iris Murdoch points out in one of her novels that it is a very strange thing the way acute attention, focused attention, is so close to going to sleep. That's one of the ways of hypnotizing: a tremendous sort of focused attention is directed upon something. So there is an acute attention, and a loss of attention.

NANCY ANDREASEN   Well, it's diversion of attention from everything out there, from pain in the body or whatever to something else.

DICK SELZER   Isn't there the reverse situation too? I'm thinking, for example, about the stigmatics and the ability to make oneself sick or develop wounds.

JO TRAUTMANN   That seems to be much easier, doesn't it?

GENE MOSS   I don't agree. I think we are constantly willing ourselves into health, and it's against that background that an illness occurs and a patient and a physician encounter one another.

JIM COWAN   This whole question of willing yourself into health in any cooperative effort between doctor and patient suggests that there are psychological resources—some people would say spiritual resources—at any rate, some tangible strengths which the patient can tap. Can we train people in this process?

JO TRAUTMANN   And the next obvious question is, do we train them partly by teaching them to read and write literature?

JIM COWAN   I think this can be done.

GENE MOSS   Let me describe my experience with Elizabeth's paper. At first encounter, it put me off because it seemed to be directing us out of an area where we have some authority and experience and capabilities, and into an area where we have none. I stopped being put off by that, although I didn't change my opinion. That is to say, Elizabeth's inviting us and others to divest ourselves of a kind of arrogance may be nothing *but* arrogance. Again and again we are confronted with the idea that we've made enormous advances in the last five, twenty, or fifty years in terms of what we understand and how we can control what we understand. In reality, I expect, we've only scratched the surface. We've only begun to understand what is the real complexity on the material level of the world around us. We've gotten a certain kind of power, but whether it amounts to much or not remains to be seen.

What you're inviting us to do, Elizabeth, is to back out of that arrogance, I think, to a very fruitful point of viewing ourselves and the things we believe and the language we use objectively. My problem is: how can we communicate about that? We're quickly going to end up as we began. We could go on citing example after example of things science can't accomplish and which maybe require some other method of perception. We have the baggage of our language, the only tool we've got to work with in our dialogue group. We've got experiences that are perhaps not irrelevant, but how can we get to the theoretical issues if language is on one hand the tool, and on the other, a barrier?

When asked to deal with magic and magical phenomena, Elizabeth, you say that Apollonian language doesn't address them well, yet you immediately go to poetic and fictive language—another sort of language. That suggests that dealing with the language disparity in a more discursive way is difficult or even impossible. Still, I'm much more at ease with this solution now, and I'm much more positive about our doing this than I was at first.

JO TRAUTMANN   Let me ask you a question, Elizabeth. Under ideal circumstances, is there a way in which we who have been very theoretical and rational about a lot of things—is there a way we could meet at some point to discuss magic and medicine? How would we go about it? Would we sit and read poetry together? Would we encounter each other in some of the ways we learned in the sixties? What would we do to begin to be receptive to this kind of subject? Or what could physicians and literary people do together to be receptive to what is obviously a long and rigorous study?

ELIZABETH SEWELL   This is to me an experimental and experiential matter. That's what my Pythagoras is all about, and the answer is still ahead of me.

JO TRAUTMANN   One of the inroads might be the subject that several of us here are interested in, that is, the study of the body in nonmedical ways. If we keep studying the body in those ways, we can take our bodies back, and then when we go to see a physician, our bodies *are* ourselves, our illnesses, our health. Up to now, when we walked into a doctor's office or were wheeled into an operating room, we gave our bodies to the doctors, together with our will, I'm afraid.

ELIZABETH SEWELL   I want to pick up one tiny thing about powers we don't use [earlier Dick had lamented the passing of powers like clairvoyance and certain olfactory and tactile capacities] and your interesting use of the word "will." I want really to pursue this business about learning to die. It's quite clear that human beings do have the capacity to will their death. We know that. I would like to learn to do so also because I think it may be necessary to point out how it's done. It's clear that those we call "simple" and "primitive" peoples have this capacity.

SEVERAL DIALOGISTS   Hm−m−m.

JO TRAUTMANN   Do you want to stop. Do you want to go to lunch before we consider Gene's paper?

ELIZABETH SEWELL   I find myself just suddenly, yes, a little tired.

GLANCES AT MADNESS AND LITERATURE
Harold Gene Moss

The relationship between insanity and literature can be explored at four points of connection.

1. *Madness in the Artist.* A phenomenon of mutual concern to the literary and medical communities, the frequency of mental illness in writers almost certainly is higher than in typical samples of the American population and almost certainly derives from a "Romantic" definition of the artist's identity, objectives, and role in society. Within this proposition—advanced by different discussions we've had so far I think—the key issue seems to be the source from which the artist's special author-

ity arises: the Romantic belief that *experience* transcending the usual inspires special insights into a truth that is exquisitely torturous to communicate. Unlike the epic narrator in classical literature, the transcendence of the Romantic poet is introverted, personal, socially dislocating and built upon living, physical experience. His ecstasy alienates the artist from society, then destroys him.

A contrast between the roles and functions of the poet in Thomas Gray's "The Bard" and Samuel Johnson's "Rasselas" (chapter 40) identifies the eighteenth century as a transitional period wherein the older, neoclassical definition of the poet as "legislator" gave way to the "romantic" role common in the twentieth century.

Writers like Sylvia Plath, Anne Sexton, and others who committed suicide are seen by a small but devoted audience in terms of their illnesses. Such audiences then seek in the artists' lives manifestations of personality that correspond to effects or methods within the art. While this critical approach is inevitable with one's popular contemporaries, it easily abuses the very complex process of artistry and the equally complex circumstances of a human life. It also runs a constant risk of circular reasoning.

Kenneth Burke's *The Philosophy of Literary Form*, a work of much wisdom, asserts the possibility that the complex of symbols in "Kubla Khan" and "The Rime of the Ancient Mariner" would yield to biographical interpretation if all the patterns of symbolic relationship in Coleridge's life were understood. Burke's promise of a detailed explication of the poems was never written, suggesting that such analysis may in fact be an impossibility.

2. *Art in Madmen.* I know nothing about the art produced by patients as part of a therapeutic program. Nancy mentioned this in passing. If it had much consequence for us, I suppose she would have said more.

3. *Art in Madness.* I gather that structuralist psychology addresses the mental patterns and organization of the insane. For various reasons, I have undertaken a program of reading in "structuralism," a program largely oriented toward literary studies, linguistics, and anthropology. I know not to what degree structuralism has proven a workable clinical method, but at a glance it seems worth investigating, particularly with the forms of mad-

ness that are dislocations of usual mental pattern rather than a general dissolution of psychic structure.

4. *Madness in Art.* Jim's essay on Lawrence and Bill's study of "spleen" identify one approach to madness in art. The basic proposition seems to be that writers of the past modified and used the science of their time. The more precise our knowledge of the use by artists of such sources, the greater our understanding and appreciation of their art. The value of such scholarship is unquestionable; it runs only one risk, namely that it may be abused by attacking the integrity of art through a reductive explanation of its objectives and methods.

Another possible approach to "madness in art" would be to find ways in which writers, acting self-consciously and fully in control of their medium, attempt to represent a disorder of mind in the work they produce. This, I believe, may be particularly revealing because the primary act of the artist touches on many of the considerations central to the mind of man and its relation to body, to sensation, to society, and to questions of life's purposes. To represent madness the artist must explicitly disorganize elements of a symbolic communication that are inherently organized if they are meaningful. It is possible that we can find some special insights into the nature of both art and madness by examining in the following pages works by several authors; my hope is that we may at once serve the interests of medicine and literature by probing the nature of "order" and "disorder" in literature. I shall attempt to begin this discussion by directing remarks to several poems—good enough to deserve serious study and short enough to be treated with some adequacy.

II

By their nature, the arts always develop a tension between order and disorder. In static arts such as painting and architecture, the disorder is rendered as a controlled tension within the static arrangement, existing also at the border, the frame, the boundary of the space given structure by the art work. In the dynamic arts, which include music, cinema, and literature, the tension is inherent in the rhythm, in the flow of images and plot which occur in temporal sequence. The media of all arts have inherent properties which regularize their use, in effect ordering the messages they may communicate. But some arts are more "rational" than others, because their media are less sensory, more dependent upon a regular system of signs and symbolic relationships.

Language is the most rational of media, the most conservative, and the most orderly. Its use as an art form depends upon a knowledge of arbitrary signification shared by author and audience. Yet, significantly, its rational basis is always threatened at the instant when an image (a reference to sensory information) becomes a metaphor (a likeness stated or implied). This act of making metaphor, I assert, is central to the art of literature and its equivalent is central to the act of comprehension constantly at work in the minds of all human beings. Thus, of all art forms, literature must strain most to represent disorder. How easily it is done in painting (Goya's *Dog Buried in Sand*), in music (Stravinsky's *Sacre du printemps*), or film (Renais's *Marienbad*).

Now the strategies used by authors to represent mental disorder in their art may be grouped into three categories: a) madness represented in characters; b) madness represented in the world surrounding sane characters; c) madness embodied in the artwork itself. A discussion and illustration of each of these strategies will reveal some fundamental and recurrent features of madness in art.

Robert Browning's monologue "Porphyria's Lover" (1836) is a fascinating study of necrophilia and the psychology of murder. It goes beyond the bizarre by the force of its utterance and by the connections Browning makes between the excess of his character and the confused social values that stand as background for those excesses. Browning's madman is the epitome of his godless age, simultaneously brutal and pathetic.

The poem opens with a surprising projection of volition into the activity of inanimate nature:

> The rain set early in tonight,
>   The sullen wind was soon awake,
> It tore the elm-tops down for spite,
>   And did its worst to vex the lake.

(ll. 1–4)

The speaker's response highlights the mental tensions behind his perception: "I listened with heart fit to break. / When glided in Porphyria" (ll. 5−6). The next 25 lines describe Porphyria's actions and motives, all of which are particularly accented by the total passivity the speaker attributes to himself. In line 31 is the reference to his first slight movement, one still restrained by uncertainty:

> Be sure I looked up at her eyes
>   Happy and proud; at last I knew
> Porphyria worshiped me: surprise
>   Made my heart swell, and still it grew
>   While I debated what to do.
>
> (ll. 31−35)

The heart "fit to break" (l. 5) becomes by line 34 swollen, "and still it grew." And his uncertainty about the volition of nature, (in ll. 2−4), of Porphyria (in ll. 6−30), and of himself (in ll. 15−16, l. 35) gives way to violence:

> I found
> A thing to do, and all her hair
>   In one long yellow string I wound
>   Three times her little throat around,
> And strangled her.
>
> (ll. 37−41)

The poem ends in three passages: the speaker's comment on the painlessness of Porphyria's death, a description of his necrophilic lovemaking, and a description of the perfect stillness that follows.

The tensions in the poem between order and disorder are both stylistic, in the rhythm of the verse, and substantive, in the actions and images developed through the speaker's mind. I'll say little about the former, noting only that the poem's metrical form is very regular, twelve stanzalike units each with five octosyllabic lines rhyming *a b a b b*. Against this regular measure, Browning employs enjambment to disorganize his basic rhythm with particularly spectacular effects at ll. 40−41 and ll. 55−56.

In substance, Browning develops the following oppositions:

Order	Disorder
Cottage	Storm
Color	Pale
Stability	Mutability
Warm	Cold
Silence	Noise

While all of these are conventional, his departures from convention reveal a special strategy. The following oppositions are *reversed* in the poem:

Order	Disorder
Sexuality	Necrophilia
Procreation	Murder
Pleasure	Pain
Preservation	Destruction

It is powerfully illustrated in the poem that these reversals are employed in the metaphoric uses of language. First, in "the sullen wind" is "awake," then in "Porphyria" "glided," and finally in the concretizing of the metaphor of orgasmic "death." *Le petit mort* becomes biological death.

In briefly summarizing Browning's strategy in the representation of madness, we should note three tactics:

1. Establishment of regular patterns in style and in substance, in the form of oppositions.
2. Variations on regular style and reversals of opposition disorder the conventional and regular.
3. Rationality gives way to ironic paradox.

In "Porphyria's Lover," the last line, "And yet God has not said a word!" explodes the final irony. The Christian paradox of eternal life through temporal death is effected by the lover. He expects God's jealousy, not God's justice.

Of the many other works of literature that represent madness in characters, one may note Shakespeare's *Hamlet*, John Dryden's *Aureng-Zebe*, Jonathan Swift's *Modest Proposal*, Edgar Allen Poe's *The Fall of the House of Usher*, and Herman Melville's *Moby Dick*. Poems by Hopkins, Donne, Blake, and other overtly religious authors represent meditative ecstasy with strategies similar to or identical with Robert Browning's, except the final paradox is pressured with meaning, not surrounded by irony.

The second category of literature—works that represent madness in the setting but not in characters—are all satires. Horace, Juvenal, and a legion of more recent satirists employ the contrast between an overt sanity in character (often the speaker of the work) and an overt insanity in the ambient setting. In writers of fiction, the names of Cervantes, Thomas Hardy, George Eliot, James Joyce, Ernest Hemingway, Joseph Heller, and Thomas Pynchon are of prime importance. Blake's "London" (1794) stands as an excellent example in this category.

> I wander thro' each charter'd street,
> Near where the charter'd Thames does flow,
> And mark in every face I meet
> Marks of weakness, marks of woe.
>
> In every cry of every Man,
> In every Infant's cry of fear,
> In every voice, in every ban
> The mind-forg'd manacles I hear.
>
> How the Chimney-sweeper's cry
> Every black'ning Church appalls;
> And the hapless Soldier's sigh
> Runs in blood down Palace walls.
>
> But most thro' midnight streets I hear
> How the youthful Harlot's curse
> Blasts the new-born Infant's tear,
> And blights with plagues the Marriage hearse.

Normative values in the poem arise from the spontaneous, the innocent, the biological, and are used to measure the rational (perhaps rationalized) over-organization of life. The industrial forms of society (in the chimney-sweeper, the soldier, the harlot) threaten to infiltrate and destroy even man's innate imaginative biological capacities.

Now "London" can be examined in relation to the strategies employed by Browning in "Porphyria":

1. *Establishment of regular patterns in style and convention-*

al oppositions in images. Blake employs a conventional four line stanza, varied only by repetition of phrases in the first stanza: "chartered" (l. 1 and l. 2); "mark" as verb (l. 3) and "Marks" as noun (l. 4); and by parallel prepositional phrases, "In every . . ." (ll. 5, 6, 7). Blake's phrase "mind-forg'd manacles" is the key to oppositions of images in the poem. He opposes the spontaneous, hence "free," against those social structures which confine and restrict: "charter'd" streets and rivers, "Palace walls," and the economic roles that imprison men and women.

2. *Reversal of conventional oppositions.* Blake reverses the conventional only once in the poem and thereby provides us with a key to the particular target of the poem's satire: "How the Chimney-sweeper's cry / Every black'ning Church appalls" (ll. 9–10).

3. *Rationality gives way to ironic paradox* with the bitter pun on "Marriage hearse" with which Blake ends. "Every black'ning Church" corrupts the mind and body of the harlot as well as the infant as well as those who ride "the Marriage hearse"—an instrument of death in life. Thus Blake's speaker, whose only actions are walking and observing, exposes the insanity of society as it appears in the ambient setting of the poem.

The third category of madness in literature is less common. The embodiment of madness in art, to make in effect a specimen of insanity, runs the risk of a total collapse of communication. Elizabeth's treatment of Lewis Carroll and others in *The Field of Nonsense* (Folcroft, 1952) suggests one method: the development of overly structured forms (in style or thought or image) wherein the reference beyond the work—the usual use of language—falls inward upon itself. Archibald MacLeish's "The End of the World" (1926) illustrates the category as it sets forth a vision of life as a circus, a strange Berkeleian world in which the attention of the spectator alone sustains the fantasy of life. Most especially, MacLeish shows us the inherent irony of a world fashioned alone from words, from the frail assumptions and conceptions we spectators make as "Quite unexpectedly the top blew off" (l. 8). And why, we may ask, does this world end?

The best answer implied in the text of the poem arises from a play between the tight sonnet form of the verse and the unexpected transformations of language use in three key passages in the first two quatrains. In l. 2 MacLeish presents us with an "armless ambidextrian"; in ll. 5–6 we are told that "the drum / Pointed"; and in ll. 6–7 MacLeish asserts that "Teeny was about to cough / In waltz-time." Added to these strange distortions of language, MacLeish gives us an equally strange sense of randomness in the exact naming of totally unexplicated characters: "Vasserot" (l. 1), "Ralph the lion" (l. 4), "Madame Sossman" (l. 5), "Teeny" (l. 6), and "Jocko" (l. 7). The combination of this false sense of concreteness and the near logic of the almost non-sense of the three passages weaves into the poem a vision of a world coming unhinged, a world vulnerable to the distractions of a confused audience, a world constructed from nothing but the passing attention of its "spectators." To put the matter simply, MacLeish fashions in the poem a spectacular vision of an insanity deep within the fabric of the poem's form and language usage.

Christopher Smart's "Jubilate Agno" (1736) might serve as yet another example. Its several hundred lines are arranged arbitrarily by first word and present us with a deluge of images to the glory of God. Scholars still debate whether the poem is art or an unhappy symptom of Smart's madness.

An alternative to MacLeish and Smart's method of handling the subject is Coleridge's "Kubla Khan" (1816), a poem composed, as its author says, "in a sort of reverie brought on by two grains of opium." The materials within the work and the history of critical response to it suggest that in fact the disorder that metaphor always brings to literature has swept beyond usual limits in this poem. The substance of the work with its special intricacy is perhaps nothing more than the vehicle of a metaphor, the tenor (the referent) having been subtracted entirely from what is written. Put more simply, the poem contains nothing but a series of provocative images, none of which are explicitly logical in their combination but all of which point generally to some scheme of meaning. Coleridge has enticed many readers to impart meaning to the poem and thus provide the missing parts of what they read as allegory.

The best response of this kind focuses on its conclusion wherein the transcendent vision of the poet both exalts him and isolates him from the society of his fellow humans:

> And all who heard should see them there,
> And all should cry, Beware! Beware!
> His flashing eyes, his floating hair!
> Weave a circle round him thrice,
> And close your eyes with holy dread,
> For he on honey-dew hath fed,
> And drunk the milk of Paradise.
>
> (ll. 48–54)

Now if this statement is seen as the poem's central concern, the patterns of thought and image in the preceding forty-seven lines may be read in relation to imagination and artistic creativity. In part, this conclusion is possible.

Oppositions include the following:

Life	*Death*
Flowing water—Liquid ("Alph, the Sacred river," l. 3 and l. 24; "mighty fountain," l. 19; and "sinuous rills," l. 8)	Still water—frozen ("sunless sea," l. 5; "lifeless ocean," l. 28; "caves of ice," ll. 36 and 47)
Creative passion ("damsel," ll. 37 ff.)	Sexual frustration ("Woman wailing," l. 16)
Peace ("gardens," l. 8)	War ("ancestral voices," l. 30)

If this were all, the poem would be wholly explicable and very dull. In fact, Coleridge folds one image into another through a process similar to metaphor but metaphor gone wild, metaphor exploding free of any rational or orderly connection between vehicle and tenor.

Reference in the poem proceeds from literal toward figurative. The first fourteen lines challenge us only with "pleasure dome" and "caverns measureless to man," both of which are fuzzy but understandable. The descriptions of the "romantic chasm" (ll. 12–16) and the origin of the river (ll. 17–29) begin to strain language:

> A savage place! as holy and enchanted
> As e'er beneath a waning moon was haunted
> By woman wailing for her demon-lover!
>
> (ll. 14–16)

To express savagery, holiness, and enchantment in terms of "waning moon," haunting, "woman wailing," and "demon-lover" is to reverse the usual relationship between vehicle and tenor. We can still follow the comparison, but the image of "romantic chasm" is more accessible than "woman wailing for her demon-lover." Similarly "ceaseless turmoil" is explained, "as if this earth in fast thick pants were breathing" and "Huge" boulders are said to have

> vaulted like rebounding hail,
> Or chaffy grain beneath the thresher's flail:
> And 'mid these dancing rocks at once and ever
> It flung up momently the sacred river.
>
> (ll. 21–24)

The violence of nature in both cases is closer to sense and experience than the "breathing" of the earth and "dancing rocks."

The force of all this is felt when, for the first time, the first-person speaker enters the poem at l. 37:

> A damsel with a dulcimer
> In a vision once I saw:
> It was an Abyssinian maid,
> And on her dulcimer she played,
> Singing of Mount Abora.
> Could I revive within me
> Her symphony and song,
> To such a deep delight 'twould win me,
> That with music loud and long,
> I would build that dome in air,
> That sunny dome! those caves of ice!
>
> (ll. 37–47)

The apparently radical shift in the poem's direction and subject gives way to the assertion with which the passage closes: "with music loud and long, / I would build that dome in air," a statement that leaves the reader breathless with the implication that all the things described—Khan, river, chasm—exist merely on a vanishing frontier of relationships between experience and imagination.

To return now to the representational strategies used by Browning and Blake, we find that madness is similarly represented by Coleridge:

1. *Establishment of regular patterns in style and conventional oppositions in images.* Regularity in versification proceeds from an alternating rhyme scheme, most regular in the first verse paragraph, least regular in ll. 37–44 where three lines with no rhyme (37, 38, and 41) and two feminine rhymes (ll. 42 and 44) appear. By the poem's end, the regularity of the opening verse paragraph is restored. As already noted, the poem's basic pattern of images follows conventional oppositions between life and death.

2. *Reversal of conventional oppositions.* Here Coleridge departs from the paradigm in that he does not reverse convention but rather combines opposed images to assert transcendence. Twice he exclaims: "A sunny pleasure-dome with caves of ice!" (l. 36). "That sunny dome! those caves of ice!" (l. 47), thus identifying the source of heightened awareness in the clash of sun and ice—life and death.

3. *Rationality gives way to ironic paradox.* The poem's last verse paragraph combines two points of view, one internal and one external. Internally, the paradoxical images, sun and ice, combine in an exalted vision. Externally, one sees the poet with "His flashing eyes, his floating hair!" (l. 50)—victim of his "vision."

I would argue that Coleridge has produced a poem that in effect embodies madness not in the characters described or in the setting depicted, but rather in its very fabric, in the images combined in special kinds of metaphors. Coleridge communicates insanity as the imaginative faculty gone wild. It surely resembles meditative and devotional poetry except that the fundamental paradox of Christianity—life through death—is replaced by paradoxical images of life in death. The insanity Coleridge expresses with the poem is the madness of artistic inspiration.

To conclude, I will merely note the special kinds of problems that occur as literature represents madness. By its nature, language is rational. Imaginative writing always develops tension between the rational and the irrational, between the orderly reference of noun to thing and the imaginative leap of metaphor. As this tension is pushed to its limits by some of our best authors—Homer in *The Iliad*, Cervantes in *Don Quixote*, Kafka in *The Trial*, Shakespeare, Blake, Keats—the result is masterpieces of the most extraordinary kind. The trick is to control the tension and to unleash its force progressively. The other arts are under a similar obligation but, because their media are less conceptual, they may communicate more directly the imaginative disorder of madness.

Gene Moss had known that madness was the chief topic upon which people from literature and medicine had "consulted" in the past. The most predictable response to this knowledge would have been, I suppose, this one: let's go on to something else, then, especially since Nancy Andreasen, who is superbly suited to discuss the topic, has already done so, and Bill Ober, a psychobiographer with an extraordinary command of the historical method and the literature which illustrates his chosen aspect of madness, has further illuminated the topic.

But Gene elected to stay with it. The dialogists were glad that he did, for it would be misleading to assume that literature and medicine is anything but a new field, even in this, its most longstanding mutual concern. By carefully spelling out the four points at which the literary and medical communities might meet upon the topic, Gene showed us that it was chiefly "Madness in the Artist" which had held our interest in the past, and secondly, "Madness in Art" in a very particular sense, helpful certainly to both communities. But Gene asserted that there was more work to be done. So he examined the methods of the artists, and the structures of the art work, doing so in a manner that would please literature's most "scientifically" inclined critics.

In short, Gene's approach was designed to appeal to both medical and literary readers, without condescending to either group, certainly without compromising the integrity of the field in which he is the expert. More than that, he explicitly stated that he hoped his conclusions would be simultaneously valuable for those who seek to elucidate the art of poetry and those who seek to help people clinically, which—considering that "clinical" help may be given at one remove as well as none—meant that he was addressing the dialogists themselves, all of us.

Although Gene had to skip over two of his four points ("Art in Madmen" and "Art in Madness") fairly quickly, their inclusion gave completeness to his assessment of the topic and provided some hints for further research—not only by the psychiatrists alone, but also with the assistance of literary people. As a matter of fact, Nancy had sent the dialogists a set of poems written by some of her patients, whose permission she had obtained prior to distributing the works.

Jo Trautmann shared with Gene Moss a concern to pay careful attention to the directions the dialogue had taken in earlier meetings. Since the group had decided that "The Body" was of common concern, she selected the life and work of Anton Chekhov in order to explore some additional aspects of the group's interest. Since the group had frequently discussed the differences between quantitative and imaginative reporting, she wrote about Chekhov's *The Island*, where that very same tension is operating, a book by an author who experienced those tensions in his life as well. Madness and self-healing were touched on; and the use of language to measure as well as to unite.

In a sense, her essay was a communication to Dick Selzer and an attempt to try to understand those in whom literature and medicine come together. There was also a specific incident in Meeting Three to which the Chekhov essay was an indirect response. At that meeting Dick had told us about an essay he had just written called "What I Saw at the Abortion."[5] What he saw was an operation to remove a six-month fetus. At the moment the needle was inserted the fetus jumped. Dick was horrified and recorded his horror, only to become, upon publication of the essay, an unwilling champion of the right-to-life groups. He claimed that as an artist he had the obligation to observe only, and he couldn't control the audience's response. But Denise, who also held that the artist didn't have the responsibility to right all communal wrongs, was intrigued at Meeting Three by her own anger as a pro-abortionist. So Jo's paper also touched on the question of whether the artist's responsibility should be to observe as clearly as possible, or whether as a humanitarian, his or her duty is to help matters more directly. Such a tension is complicated when both roles are played by the doctor, who is committed to remaining "objective."

Jo was trying to respond to previous discussions and to push the group further through the use of the word *prison*, both as reality and as metaphor. In this way she hoped not only to understand Chekhov better, but to provide everyone with a metaphoric key (so shall prison be turned into key) by which to deal with serious, chronic illness and early death.

DOCTOR CHEKHOV'S PRISON

Joanne Trautmann

Anton Chekhov wrote five major plays and hundreds of stories. Thousands of his letters have survived. At least one good biography has appeared in English. In spite of all this material, it is hard to derive a composite picture of him as a public and private man. Yet I feel we must try, for he was an artist and a doctor—a great artist and a doctor.

When I first arrived at the Medical Center, I almost ritualistically hung pictures of Williams and Chekhov, in order that they might serve as Presences while I slowly reread each of them in my peripherally medical environment. First Dr. Williams in this way yielded new pleasures and significance, and now I turn to Chekhov, hearing as I do Denise's voice from the tape of our first hour's meeting sharply asking why "The Doctor as Writer" was on our list of potential subjects, why indeed the claim was made that this subject might somehow sum up the others, when to her it seemed the most irrelevant of all; and remembering my own haughty line, written elsewhere, to the effect that there were surely less superficial subjects than Williams and Chekhov for those of us interested in "literature and medicine." Still, I believe that we as a group must try out this subject, perhaps laying it to rest as irrelevant or superficial, but perhaps, as I suspect, finding in Chekhov something of very special value for those people in medicine and in literature who look to each other's disciplines for insights. This is dialogue as discovery.

In our conversations we can't concentrate solely on either the art or the man because whatever Chekhov can offer to our situation becomes evident through both his literary works and his life as a medical professional, as well as through his comments on the two as they coexisted. It would indeed be rather superficial, though not without value to be sure, to survey here the portraits of doctors drawn by Chekhov in several of his stories and most of his major plays. Likewise to consider his fictional explorations of medical matters like disease and suffering (and there is such a lot of both in this Russian) would be satisfying to a degree, but finally predictable. Coming at the subject from an exclusively biographical angle—for example, comparing his 1884 letter to Nikolay Leikin about an autopsy with the resulting story of 1885, "The Dead Body"—is not quite the point either. No, we must use all the available approaches, somehow combining them if possible.

Of course critics and biographers of Chekhov have dealt often with this matter of the writer who is also a doctor who is also a writer, and it might be useful to put out on our examining table a brief summary of the stands taken in the past. They seem to have been an obvious and complacent lot. (I know this because I have confidently repeated all of them in lectures!) Anton Chekhov, it is said, could write realistically about such an astonishing variety of people—provincial intellectuals, soldiers, peasants, men, women, and children of all sorts—because as a doctor he treated such a variety of people. He had admirable tolerance for even the vilest of characters because he knew that human suffering is universal. Though he had compassion for almost every one of his characters ("The author must be humane to the tips of his fingernails," he wrote to Yelena Shavrova), he kept his distance because as a doctor he quite naturally turned his training in clinical detachment into an aesthetic theory about observer objectivity ("The writer ought not to judge his characters or what they say, but be only an unbiased witness"). He knew a good deal about mental and physical disease, but he never in his art lost sight of the patient.

True, no doubt, all more-or-less true, but many things about this doctor-writer still escape us, and I'd like to pursue just one main idea, together with some oblique references to our previous discussions, in an attempt to make the man and his work a bit clearer, and to set out some issues I'd like to discuss.

Consistent with his theories about authorial objectivity, Chekhov hides himself so carefully in his stories and plays—normally spreading his identity throughout all his characters, rather than choosing one for his representative—that biographical criticism, a risk at the best of times, is foolhardy in Chekhov's case. But there is one work in which this private man shows himself. I turn to it because the work seems to be central to Chekhov's world view and therefore central to his artistic, medical, and more directly personal concerns. I refer to Chekhov's book-length study called *The Island: A Journey to Sakhalin.*[6]

For those unfamiliar with the work, I will briefly describe and evaluate *The Island.* In the first place, it confounds all attempts to fit it into a genre, which is probably to its credit, and is usually called simply "nonfiction." It is, among other things, a sociological and medical study of penology—for Sakhalin was the place of exile for serious criminals—a portrait of a depressed people, and a travel diary. Though his letters detail the harsh six-thousand-mile journey from Moscow through Siberia to this narrow six-hundred-mile-long island afloat in the Sea of Okhotsk north of Japan, the book itself begins with the traveller's arrival in the Eastern port city of Nikolayevsk, on the River Amur, and carries him through his three months on the island. During that time he conducts singlehandedly a census of the inhabitants, filling out his personally devised census cards, he claims, for 10,000 settlers. Like a scientific anthropologist, he relies on this method to get statistical data, with which he loads his book; at the same time, like a humanistic anthropologist, he merely uses such easy-to-answer factual questions—what is your religion? when did you arrive? do you receive assistance?—to get closer to the people he was interviewing, or, as Chekhov puts it, "to gain impressions through the recording process itself." He proceeds from prison to prison, hut to hut, settlement to settlement, interviewing the nonpolitical convicts, the ex-convicts who were not yet allowed to leave the island for Russia, and the "free" people— spouses, children—who accompanied them. Everywhere he narrates the history of the place, complete with admirably scholarly apparatus, and describes, statistically when possible, the prevailing conditions: "It has ninety inhabitants, sixty-three males and twenty-seven females; fifty-two homesteaders." All of this "science" is interspersed with little Chekhovian vignettes and characters—a doctor who looks like Ibsen, a police official who writes fiction and takes Chekhov to an unspeakable brothel, a five-year-old girl who clings to her father's chains, people whose bizarre surnames mean "Mr. Nameless," "Mr. Countryless," and "Mr. Unremembered."

The combined tone is strange and to me not very satisfactory. It is best called reportage, I suppose, but little judgments break out here and there—"he is suffering"; "when such a man stands before you in a pitifully worn jacket, you do not think of his crime." They are *little* judgments, however, and therefore merely distracting. As Robert Payne, who has introduced *The Island*, points out, there is one incident which is described with "no detachment,"[7] and that is in Derbinskoye when Chekhov observes rain-soaked, mud-covered prisoners, pleading to be sent to the hospital and trying to act out in mime what their illnesses were. Remembering the mysterious moans as he had fallen asleep the night before, Chekhov writes, "My nightmare seemed to be continuing. . . . I felt that I saw before me the extreme limits of man's degradation, lower than which he cannot go." But this sort of judgment is rare in the book, maybe unique, and on the whole we have this distancing, not so much like the sort of artistic objectivity noticed by all readers of his stories, nor entirely a neat, clear researcher's report either, but a kind of horrifying—and here my prejudices will show—*sociological* distancing, a seemingly fraudulent caring, though we know that Chekhov cared deeply. The last chapter is the oddest of all. Its subject is "Diseases and Mortality of the Convict Population." There are remnants of the vaguely novelistic rendering seen earlier: "I become convinced during my short visit to the island that colds play the main role in the etiology of this illness, those who are stricken being people who work in the taiga in cold and raw weather and who sleep under the open sky. People suffering from this illness are most frequently seen on roadwork and on new settlement sites. This is veritable *febris sachalinensis*." But most of the chapter is straightforward recording of facts, the number of scurvy cases in 1889, the deaths from syphilis, that sort of thing. And the four-hundred-page book ends abruptly in a scholarly parenthesis: "Convict women are usually permitted one and a half years to breast-feed their children. (*Code on Convicts,* Article 297, 1890 edition.)"

Part of the problem with the book's tone is attributable to Chekhov's inexperience with this style of writing. He wanted to be thought a scholar. He had months of trouble putting the book together after he got home. And one sees, of course, that he consciously chooses the method of speaking the facts and letting the horrors speak for themselves. But the tone and the unsatisfactory mix are not entirely explained in this way. I'm convinced that the other part of the explanation is related to Chekhov's attitude towards the subject itself. After three months of plodding about the island like a scholarly scientist, he exhales his true attitude in the freedom of a letter to his friend Suvorin: "As long as I was staying in Sakhalin, I only felt a certain bitterness in my innards, as if from rancid butter; but now, in retrospect, the island seems to me a perfect hell" (9 December 1890).[8] Understandably so, for Sakhalin in its very existence stood for the concept of imprisonment, and everywhere Chekhov travelled on the cut-off bit of land, he encountered wretched examples of the loss of freedom that was not only his foremost intellectual *bête noir*, but also, as I hope to demonstrate, the most looming nightmare of his soul and body.

No wonder that, faced with months of living within a giant prison, where most of the people he encountered began their talk of the time past with "When I was free . . . ," and when the captain of the ship hired to bring new prisoners to the island said, "We are the prisoners, not the convicts," and when even the humor cannot escape prison imagery ("'Why are your pig and rooster tied up?' I asked a householder. 'In our Sakhalin everything is chained,' he replied jokingly.")—no wonder that a man like Chekhov sees his journey to Sakhalin as hellish and in the writing of *The Island* handles his horror so badly.

Why then did he make this journey? That is a question that he himself answers several times in his letters, constantly shifting his explanations, because clearly he was not entirely sure, but I am convinced that the truest motive was his compulsion to face in reality the most profound metaphor of his life, the prison, and to enact, if possible, the sort of release that neither his writing nor his medicine could give him. Put another way, he seems to have been called on a venture into hell for his soul's sake (he writes in passing to one friend that he may not return), and instead of sending another fictional envoy, he goes this time himself.

Although he was only thirty years old when he journeyed to Sakhalin, Chekhov was already an important writer and had, in fact, written most of the stories for which he is still famous. Sakhalin was therefore a culmination of years of writing about freedom and its loss, a theme that had its original inspiration in the facts of Chekhov's childhood. His grandfather was a serf who bought the freedom of his family, but not soon enough for Chekhov's provincial father to escape the petty mentality of the slave, and in his turn he played the tyrant to his children, a fact Chekhov emphasizes in a letter to his brother Aleksandr: "I ask you to recall that despotism and lying ruined your mother's life. Despotism and lying mangled our childhood . . ." (2 January 1889). In two other well-known letters he speaks of what freedom means to him, and why. To Aleksey Pleshcheyev he writes on 4 October 1888: "My holy of holies is the human body, health, intelligence, talent, inspiration, love and absolute freedom." And to Suvorin, he suggests this story outline, obviously derived from his own life:

> Write a story, do, about a young man, the son of a serf, a former grocery boy, a choir singer, a high school pupil and university student, brought up to respect rank, to kiss the hands of priests, to truckle to the ideas of others—a young man who expressed thanks for every piece of bread, who was whipped many times, who went out without galoshes to do his tutoring, who used his fists, tortured animals, was fond of dining with rich relatives, was a hypocrite in his dealings with God and men, needlessly, solely out of a realization of his own insignificance— write how this young man squeezes the slave out of himself, drop by drop, and how, on awaking one fine morning, he feels that the blood coursing through his veins is no longer that of a slave but that of a real human being. (7 January 1889)

With his imagination this man, free now as he thinks, relives over and over in his fiction the time of bondage. Occasionally he speaks both directly and metaphorically of the prison, as in "Daydreams" (1886), which starts out as the story of two country constables leading a tramp to the local magistrate, but ends as the story of three prisoners being led absolutely nowhere, but led nonetheless by the need to go on merely because there is a road. The landscape is itself a nightmarish prison with ever receding but always present walls: "There is an impenetrable wall of white fog. They walk on and on, but the ground remains the same, the wall is no nearer, and the patch is the same." The tramp, who will not give his name (cf. Sakhalin's "Mr. Nameless," "Mr. Unremembered," and "Mr. Countryless"—grim realizations of this earlier tale), reveals that he is a runaway convict, sentenced to hard labor, which he describes as being "like a lobster in a basket: there's crowding, crushing, jostling, no room to breathe; it's plain hell." He dreams now of being exiled to Eastern Siberia, and envisions himself living in "more free space," with great numbers of fish and game, fearfully steep river banks, huge trees—all in vivid contrast to the "impassable autumn mud," a fact which evidently spurs the constables to "picture to themselves a free life such as they have never lived; whether they vaguely remember scenes from stories heard long ago or whether they have inherited notions of a free life from remote free ancestors with their flesh and blood, God alone knows!" But the constables cannot sustain their dreams, nor even allow the tramp his, naïve as they know it to be, so long as it contrasts so obviously with their common lot. They brutally remind the sickly tramp of another sort of prison—you'll never get to Siberia, they tell him; they'll put you in a hospital, and you'll die—and the story ends by turning back onto itself: "The tramp is more hunched than before, and his hands are thrust deeper into his sleeves."

More commonly, Chekhov writes without direct reference to a place called a prison, but the sense of absolute confinement is there nonetheless, sometimes caused by society, occasionally by a sort of cosmic jailer, most often by forces excreted from ourselves, including disease, both physical and, especially, mental. In fact, in Chekhov's mature stories very few people escape, to Moscow or anywhere else. In "Gooseberries" the talk is of "oppression" even at the sight of happy men, especially as they are seen through windows in their separate little houses having tea with their families, when they should be out fighting for freedom for the downtrodden, against the time when trouble will come to themselves. In "Peasants" a dozen people, old and young, crowd in upon each other in a small cabin, and to this hut comes the ill Nikolay, exiled from Moscow and from freedom. "In the Cart" introduces an underpaid, overworked, and utterly alone provincial school-mistress, who dreams for one moment of happiness with a handsome neighbor, whom she cannot meet on equal terms, and then the "barrier" slowly rises again. "The Name-Day Party" is about an intelligent young wife trapped by her stupid neighbors, her own jealousy and hysteria, and finally by her pregnancy and grief, until not only her body, but her entire life seems permeated by chloroform. The little boy in "Vanka" writes piteously to his grandfather to fetch him away from the man to whom he has been apprenticed and who treats him precisely like a slave, but the letter with no address hasn't a chance of reaching the outside world. The grief-stricken father in "Misery" lives in solitary confinement. And in Chekhov's fullest fictional statement about medical matters, the remarkable "Ward 6," the doctor comes to view the mad ward as just another prison, and the question of who's in and who's out as one of chance, which prepares the way for the final twist, wherein the doctor ends as an incarcerated, brutalized inmate in his own hospital. (That a couple of these stories were written after the Sakhalin journey of 1890 is a point to which I will return later.)

Chekhov, the slave who had become a real human being, thus reexperienced the loss of freedom often through his fictional creations, until he was in danger of being oppressed again himself. It was all very well to write to Suvorin about the limitations of an artist's responsibility: "It seems to me that it is not the task of fiction writers to solve such problems as God, pessimism, etc. . . . It is time for writers, particularly artists, to confess that in this world you cannot make head or tail of anything," to maintain that artists must only observe and depict matters accurately, and nothing more (30 May 1888). But still there came to the normally cheerful man from time to time moments of gloom, anxiety, and despair, such as his characters experience. "My soul," he writes to Suvorin, "is subject to a kind of stagnation" (4 May 1889). In these moods he regretted that as an artist he could do little actively to alleviate major suffering.

In the story called "An Attack of Nerves" (1888) he has written about this impasse in both a realistic and allegorical fashion. Three students—one a student at the Moscow School of Painting, referred to throughout the story as "the artist"—spend a night carousing on the city's street of prostitution. The "law student," whose talent is for "humanity," possesses "an extraordinarily fine delicate scent for pain in general." After the visit to the brothels, where the law student has discovered not awareness of sin and hope of salvation, but only vulgar taste, he castigates his friend the artist for not acting on his artistic knowledge of the prostitutes to rescue them. Art, he declares, tells the artist that the women are morally dead years before they actually die, and he attacks the student of art for buying these women, then going freely on his way, imagining that he has the right to call himself an artist. But the artist either cannot or refuses to accept the challenge, replying that this sort of vicious attack on a friend is more immoral than all the vice in the brothels and advising the law student: "'If it is loathsome, observe it! Do you understand? Observe!'" So the artist fails to act. He leaves the equally ineffectual law student standing in a dark suffocating snowfall, similar to the scene at the end of another great work about the loss of freedom, James Joyce's *Dubliners*: "He felt frightened of the darkness of the snow which was falling in heavy flakes on the ground and seemed as though it would cover up the whole world."

But there are *three* students, the third being a student of that actively helping discipline, medicine. Alas, this young man, too, is unable or unwilling to seek release for the women, though his science tells him (says the lawyer) that all the prostitutes die prematurely of consumption or some other disease. To this, the medical student replies: "'We human beings do murder each other. . . . It's immoral, of course, but philosophizing won't help it.'" And "'One must take an objective view of things.'" Medicine also fails.

Whereupon the law student has "an attack of nerves," the sort of breakdown which Chekhov, who sometimes expressed the desire to be a psychiatrist, prided himself on being able to depict accurately. Several situations, both appalling and amusing, follow, but the only matter which need concern us at the moment is the tortured law student's conclusion that "Art and science are of no use here, that is clear. . . . The only way out of it is missionary work."

In something of the same spirit Chekhov, dissatisfied with both art and medicine, planned his missionary trip to Sakhalin. On 15 February 1890, he writes to Pleshcheyev, "In the head and on paper nothing but Sakhalin. Mania. *Mania Sakhalinosa.*"

Not that his attitude toward either of his professions had become totally negative. In fact, one of the motives he announces for his journey is to "pay off some of my debt to medicine, toward which . . . I have behaved like a pig" (to Suvorin, 9 March 1890). *The Island*'s abrupt and statistically filled last chapter, to which I have already referred, is part of his repayment, as is his hope that the book will influence reform for the ill and suffering prisoners. But Chekhov's medicine, like his art, had been weighing him down, requiring him, again like his art, to relive with nightmarish regularity his position as witness of life's prisons: suffering, disease, death. From an optimistic beginning—"I'll immerse myself in medicine, which offers a salvation" (to A. P. Chekhov, 13 May 1883)—Chekhov came to think of medicine as pulling him in a different direction from literature: "the saw about chasing two hares ["chase two hares, and you catch neither"—Russian proverb] has robbed no one of more sleep than me" (to D. V. Grigorovich, 28 March 1886); and finally to see it as something very like a restraining garment and himself as a slave, as in these lines to a friend: "Usually, when those in the household . . . are taking 'all measures' and straining every nerve, the doctor sits there and looks like a fool, discouraged, dismally ashamed of himself and his science and trying to preserve outward composure . . . Physicians go through loathsome days and hours." And this comment, sharply reminiscent of that existential serf, Kafka's "Country Doctor": "My soul is tired. Tedium. Not to belong to one's own self, to think only of diarrhea, to be startled of nights by the barking of watchdogs and knocking at the gate (have they come to fetch me?), to be driving repulsive nags over unknown roads."

Still, these frustrations must have been minor compared to

the nightmare of attending his brother Nikolay as he lay trapped in that most solid of prisons, the diseased body, knowing that he, the doctor, could do nothing to free his beloved patient of the absolutely despotic tuberculosis and typhus, and seeing him lowered into the final prison of the grave. This occurred just before Chekhov determined to journey to Sakhalin.

A cosmic wasteland, a society repressive in politics and culture—thrust through with tedium and cruelty—the artistic impasse, the diseased bodies of patients, his brother's grave: these metaphorical but increasingly claustrophobic prisons Chekhov took with him to encounter the actual prison which he must have known would confirm the worst he knew of life.

To all this we must add recognition of a still tighter, more crushing, more breathless cell, denying it until the last moment, as Chekhov did. For the fact of the matter is that when he went to Sakhalin, the doctor was already ill. Since December 1889, he had been spitting blood—from his throat, he told himself, not from his lungs like Nikolay. But of course it was tuberculosis, and he would later see the trip across Siberia as resembling "a severe, lingering illness," oppressive in the extreme (to Leontyev-Shcheglov, 10 December 1890). While on the journey he sends this admission to his sister: "[the blood] caused me to be despondent and exposed me to dismal thoughts."

Having brought my man thus burdened to this "perfect hell," as he calls it, I suppose I must bring him back, but the return is almost more dangerous for his chronicler than it was for Chekhov. Whatever the temptation to hover over his assertion that though the island of Sakhalin was hell, the island of Ceylon, at which he stopped on the return, was paradise—I must not give in. I must most certainly not linger over the possibility of calling his post-Sakhalin stories purgatorial. When Chekhov writes that "the devil only knows" what happened to him on Sakhalin, I must assume he is employing linguistic convention!

The truth is that Chekhov came back to Russia, wrote several more splendid stories, many of them, like "Gooseberries" and "Ward 6," still oppressive with prison imagery; that he continued to find the practice of medicine to some extent enslaving; that though he turned increasingly to the less claustrophic form of the drama, even there his themes were often the old ones; that far from returning as a triumphant hero, Chekhov found himself growing a pot belly and new hemorrhoids; that he became sicker and sicker, married late, spending his honeymoon in a sanatorium, and died at the age of forty-four.

The truth is also that having been compelled once to push himself to the limits of his imagination and strength and fears, something pushed him beyond his limits, and he was for a brief time "enchanted" (a word he uses in writing of the journey to Leontyev-Shcheglov), a condition that enabled him to write immediately upon his return the story of "Gusev," a tale of terrifying incarceration, but with a perfectly astonishing ending, in which the normally earthbound Doctor Chekhov turns magician.

The central event is a brave one for Chekhov to undertake at this time: the slow dying from consumption of a poor delirious sailor. Lying in the ship's infirmary with several other very ill men—including the educated and bitter Pavel Ivanych—Gusev drifts in and out of feverish memories of his family. He cannot understand Pavel Ivanych's cynical statements about the diseased poor, expressed in language natural to one who has just traversed Sakhalin: "The doctors put you on the steamer to get rid of you. They got tired of bothering with you, cattle . . . You don't pay them any money, you are a nuisance, and you spoil their statistics with your deaths." But he does register the deaths around him: first a soldier's, then Pavel Ivanych's. Finally Gusev too dies, almost unnoticeably, with hardly a break in the narrative, and with no obvious changing in point of view: "He sleeps for two days and on the third at noon two sailors come down and carry him out of the infirmary. He is sewn up in a sackcloth. . . ." The result is that when Chekhov follows Gusev's funeral details, we have the sense that he is still somehow alive—still real, certainly. So it is with increasing claustrophobic horror that we follow Gusev's besacked, weighted body, down, down into the sea, until it encounters a shark, and we cannot prevent our imaginations from seizing upon the few details we are given and rushing forward with them to the awful end—perhaps the most vivid view of the prison which Chekhov has ever written. Directly above this action, however, and simultaneously with it, the sky is coloring gorgeously. Shafts of color are streaking across the spaces. The ocean which has just gobbled up its prisoner can only momentarily defend against this expansiveness: "Looking at this magnificent enchanting sky, the ocean frowns at first, but soon it, too, takes on tender, joyous, passionate colors for which it is hard to find a name in the language of men." Thus is Doctor Chekhov's prison transcended for the moment.

That it was Gene Moss's and Jo Trautmann's essays which were central to Meeting Four enabled the dialogists to consider side by side the work of the two members who had spent the most time attempting to introduce literary methods into the medical school culture. The tapes of the discussions of these two papers show that the group was decidedly calmer—due to a number of factors, including the smaller size of the group (Ober, Levertov, and Lawson were absent). Perhaps the papers in themselves simply didn't excite as much thought for some members. But perhaps also the dialogists heard essays at this point which came from two who were a little more used to adjusting to the sort of medical-literary confrontations the group had wrestled with in previous meetings. Certainly a close look at Gene's and Jo's papers show that they were utilizing literature-and-medicine methodologies, fully aware of all the attendant dangers: being untrue to the integrity of literary methods and literature itself in attempts to meet on another discipline's ground; misvaluing medicine's interests in, for example, science and the scientific method; and being dismissed by both literary and medical people as simplistic.

But if the dialogists went home that spring in a calmer, even self-congratulatory mood, it was not lasting. In the summer Denise Levertov wrote a letter denying the value of the dialogue for her. With that letter in hand, and looking forward to Denise's paper, the freshly bestirred dialogists anticipated the fifth and last meeting.

MEETING FIVE

Necessary, Unnecessary
Journeys
The Concluding Steps

LETTER FROM DENISE LEVERTOV, 17 July 1976

What subjects would I wish to "deal with under ideal circumstances (i.e., all the time in the world, all the brains in the world!)?"[1] Well . . . assuming that, despite the expansive parenthesis, the question is still attached to our theme of Literature and Medicine, I have to admit that, if I've learned one thing from our meetings it is that as a poet I find all of our discussions totally irrelevant. Do I, in my other, overlapping role as a university teacher, find them equally useless? Again, I must admit I do. If we were actually down to the brass tacks of curriculum planning for pre-med and med school students, then I might have felt we were engaged in useful work (supposing us to be in a position from which our proposals might actually be adopted by some educational institution). As it is, I had come, by the end of our Florida meeting, to a distinct realization that we were indulging—at considerable monetary expense to a foundation and expense of time to ourselves (and small financial profit)—in a social activity: matching wits and words in a good-humored companionship. An innocent way to spend an occasional weekend, but of benefit to no one but ourselves. If I were a novelist I might have utilized some of this scene for my own purposes; as a poet, I would have been better employed elsewhere; as a social being I enjoyed the good company. Registration procedures at

Tufts (Spring preregistration for fall courses, necessitating my presence as a Freshman advisor and to interview applicants for my own courses) made it impossible for me to attend the fourth weekend but I doubt whether it would have changed my feeling that our symposia floated on hot air. My intention is to attend the fifth and last meeting nevertheless—partly to see everyone once more, and partly to give the whole project the benefit of the doubt: have we in fact done anything worth doing? Have I been blind and stupid not to see it? Will some illumination still occur which will reveal to me what all this has been about?

However, perhaps that parenthetical clause was meant to convey that the question was not confined to our "theme," but referred to what one would like best to discuss from a wide-open range of topics, given ample time and a sort of superbrains trust? In that case, I might say, "How to get rid of the giant corporations and the Pentagon and establish anarchocommunism without a bloody holocaust?" And even then I'd say, "But I only want to hear it talked about if the talk can lead directly to some effective action." More modestly, I'd be interested in discussions of how to raise the level of real literacy in the U.S.; or of how to confront and combat academic racism (has anyone else noted the conspicuous absence of any black and third world people from our group?). As a poet *per se* I do not feel a need for any formal discussions at all, however—I'd much sooner simply read, look, live, and go on doing my art (being an earthworm as that poem says). Even the informal conversations one has with one's peers on matters of craft and process, though enjoyable, are not essential unless occasionally one needs that particular stimulus.

I'm sorry to be so discouraging about all this, but those are honestly my conclusions. I embarked on the Literature and Medicine project in good faith—unsure of what I could contribute, but expecting to learn something from others, and that the group as a whole would achieve something of general value. In the event, I experienced social pleasure but do not feel I learned anything scientific, and as for the group's collectible achievement, it will presumably be manifested in the published papers; but would those writings be substantially different if we had not had these weekend conferences—i.e., were our journeys really necessary?

17 September 1976

JO TRAUTMANN   This letter depressed me, for as a member of the group I have had my frustrations, too, but finally it makes me combative, like Denise, in an affectionate way.

DENISE LEVERTOV *(laughing)*   You got pissed off, right?

JO TRAUTMANN   At some stage, yes. I can definitely identify a pissed-off stage somewhere in the middle of my other emotions!

MARY STEPHENS   Contrary to what you say in the first paragraph, Denise, I felt that the real value of this dialogue was that we were *not* doing curriculum planning. I think it's important in curriculum planning not to start at that point, because you get locked up in prerequisites and all those technical things, but to talk about the theoretical bases of what you might find in a course. I personally believe that from listening in on these discussions I have picked up a lot I could use in courses.

JO TRAUTMANN   I heartily endorse what Mary has said. All along, some members of this group, Bill in particular, have urged us to produce reading lists, and I have held the line against this, not only for the reason Mary gives, but also because as a teacher, I don't really want someone else to hand me a reading list. Denise says in her letter that we might as well not have met, that we could have sent each other papers. I feel that way about a reading list, and in fact have, in writing that long annotated bibliography, already done something of the sort.

DENISE LEVERTOV   I didn't mean mailing each other papers. I meant that I wonder whether the book of essays or whatever we produce will really come out of the meetings. The meetings are fun (otherwise I wouldn't be here), but is there any direct relationship between our meetings and whatever this end product is going to be?

BILL OBER   You have to interact with people in a face-to-face way. Until you actually meet people and see what they look like and get the tone of their voice, you don't really know what you're doing.

140

JIM COWAN   I think Denise was suggesting by using the word "social" in a denigrating way—

DENISE LEVERTOV   I should have said "conviviality," and I would never denigrate conviviality.

JIM COWAN   But I thought you were suggesting that this was not of genuine intellectual and professional value to the participants, and I disagree. Of course we have had "social" times, but the whole idea of a dialogue (I'm thinking of Bill's "face-to-face" statement) is that people say things and that other people respond to them, and then the first person speaks again. You have the pressure of the entire group. And while I might, if requested by an editor to do so, have written a paper of some sort on literature and medicine, it would not have been the papers I did write. I would not have taken that form if I were not trying to express myself to the other members of the group in response to things that have come up here. The real value for me professionally was an expansion of consciousness. Now you say that as a poet you haven't been changed. I simply can't believe that you haven't been altered in some way.

DENISE LEVERTOV   Of course in principle one is altering all the time, but our particular subject, and the discussion of it, has not altered me profoundly. It would be fraudulent to say so.

JIM COWAN   Let me speak more personally. I often go to professional meetings, such as those of the Modern Language Association. But there is not a forum at these meetings where you sit down and participate with your intellectual peers, people who have ideas different from your accustomed ideas. That's one of the reasons this was valuable for me. At our home universities, we are in competition with people with whom we might otherwise communicate. But I am not your competitor, so there can be a much freer exchange between us. In my case it has had direct professional results. After I presented my paper, Bill Ober wrote me a letter in which he listed some things I needed to do in order to understand what Lawrence is doing in his neuroanatomy theory. I intend to follow up these leads when I edit the new edition of *Fantasia of the Unconscious* and *Psychoanalysis and the Unconscious*. I also think the dialogue has affected my teaching. I might never devise a medical school curriculum, but it will affect my teaching of undergraduate humanities courses.

DENISE LEVERTOV   That's great, but what happened to you was a fortunate accident.

DICK SELZER   I am quite sure that coming here did not make me a better surgeon, as it did not make you a better poet. Beyond that, I know I have changed. For one thing I have met all of you, which I find an enriching experience. And I have been reading—I have read every single thing any of you has recommended to me. The group has made me a better teacher, not just a better writer, which I think it also did, but a better teacher. I teach surgery as one of the humanities, and found this experience a rich lode to mine and pass on to my students. I have one other point to make: I guess I wasn't expecting a "product," something you could pick up and put down. I expected exactly what has happened, that I would meet all of you and that we would talk without being shy.

DENISE LEVERTOV   It still seems to me false to pretend that we have an essential theme because we could have been talking about *anything* and would have produced the kind of result that is being spoken about here. Perhaps if our influence goes beyond these meetings, it will be the rings in the pool made because of our personal gratification, of which Jim and Dick have spoken.

NANCY ANDREASEN   But people are also saying that the dialogue had redeeming social value in more than the conviviality sense. They are saying that they have taken a great deal from this group which they will pour back into their students and society in general. You are saying you haven't gotten as much out of it to pour back in. But even if that is so, you have had another function very clearly in that you have given people something to pour back in. So your coming here has not been useless.

DENISE LEVERTOV   Well, if everybody feels that they've really gotten something out of it and that what they have gotten out of it is going to affect other people because of the way they have been affected, that there is going to be a chain reaction, then I take back my strictures on the whole thing.

NANCY ANDREASEN   And I think the title is relevant because if it were not for "literature and medicine," we would not be here.

JO TRAUTMANN   Let's concentrate on that for a minute. Al, you read Denise's letter as a call to define what we did, and are still doing in this meeting. That was one of the ways I also read the letter, especially in light of the way it echoed frustrations I have had. Perhaps I had imagined that early on we would say, "Yes, there is a field called Literature and Medicine, and these are its sub-topics." Whereas what the Institute asked us to do was to give it some statements on the state of the art, and we have done that, Ladies and Gentlemen! Denise, your statement is central to that task. Can we read your letter as saying that there isn't a field called literature and medicine? Are we back to what someone stated at the beginning? That we can link anything and anything else, but that it's illogical to expect "and" to link the two substantively? But as you answer this question, I ask you to look around the table and remind your-selves of what each person wrote for these discussions on the subject of literature and medicine. We have made statements. They may require a little shaping, but we have made them, I think. Up to this point, the dialogue has not gone as smoothly as the Institute's concurrent dialogues between history and medicine or even social science and medicine,[2] because we haven't the tradition those linked disciplines have, but why would we expect or even want the process to go smoothly? It's true that we have defined "literature" rather broadly. Some-times it has gone over into philosophy or religion, sometimes into myth or history. Sometimes we've talked about it as art, sometimes as a social agent. And I think that's all right. That, in fact, is one of our statements to the Institute. Literature in this group has been treated broadly. When you put "literature" together with "medicine," literature apparently becomes a broader discipline, as we have seen here.

IAN LAWSON   I would like to say several things in response to
Denise's letter. First, I certainly found these dialogues hard
work. And while I realize that the sense of doing hard work is
not justification for that work, I think it applies. And I have
observed hard work being done: the length of hours spent, the
intensity of the debate, the emotional exhaustion which all of
us have felt from time to time.

In terms of immediate productivity, has it changed me? I
don't look for profound changes in terms of outlets. I do think
it will change the style in which some things in my life might
be done because I happen to think there is a certain magic
about process, and that the common or garden arrangements
that we take for granted are actually not so common. We may
not change the Ultimates at all; indeed the Ultimates are un-
changeable anyway. We are all agreed on what truth is. It's the
sort of day-by-day details of truth that we have to work out,
and I think most of us would agree this series of conferences
has helped that process. I thought our dialogues were not necessarily meant to result in a substantial program or curricula,
but were an experiment in the interfacing of two disciplines.
The papers were the occasions for the interface. We had to talk
about something, so we created subjects. But it was to be the
nature of that interaction and the mutual intelligibility, provided we could arrive at it, that was to be the main interest,
not the subject itself. We have fulfilled our mandate.

But to consider the product: I think Denise's question is
properly put. We have to arrive at some conclusions, if only to
spare another group of people going through the same experience. First of all, we might say something with regard to
the difficulties of attaining mutual intelligibility. Surely we
should also be able to say something about the way in which
literature should be represented in proposed divisions of humanities within medical schools. Thirdly, for future research
and debate in interdisciplinary studies, we could suggest a
good range of specialized work. I think we should pass some
judgment about the numbers and lengths of meetings (I myself think it has taken this long to deal with a subject so complex). And I think we ought to be able to say a good deal about

the process. What have we learned about the nitty-gritty of getting a group like this to communicate with each other? I'd also like to say that collegiate fellowship at a national level is part of the job for you full-time academics.

As regards conceptual enlargement, I have a whole list of topics in which my concepts have been materially changed. For instance, I was just looking back on my notes about Gene Moss's paper: when is a metaphor operating as a metaphor, and when is it concealing inconsistencies that are damaging? That's a very operational problem for me. I would also like to say that I had to produce a paper that I would certainly not have produced, poor as it may be, anywhere else but here. Actually, the dialogue has been of some benefit to the job I now hold: that is, how do I listen fairly to people whose skills I will never match, whose disciplines I can't possibly understand to the depth they do, but, in my own role, whose working operations I can influence and restrict? That's actually quite a modern problem; actually, the administrative problem.

Still, Denise, I don't think we ought to try to persuade you that your report is anything other than legitimate or in fact quite proper. I think there should be people in a group like ours who at the end of it say, "In my particular situation, the usefulness of this meeting was limited by the following facts," which they would then list in order to be useful to people who attempt this kind of dialogue the next time.

O TRAUTMANN   I am very grateful for your letter. It has focused for us, as Bill's remarks often focus, the problems we have faced. But I must say that I am also personally disappointed. I wanted you to be here partly because you seem to me to have reached some kind of balance between your need to be a private poet and your need to address social problems—specifically the Vietnamese War. And I thought, "All right, the war is more or less over and here's another sort of battleground, in a sense: here's medicine in some trouble, being attacked on the grounds of dehumanization, among other things, and perhaps Denise would be very interested in this new social problem." Obviously you *were* interested for a time.

DENISE LEVERTOV   Perhaps if we had addressed the social aspects more directly and more often, I would have gotten out
my battle-axe.

NANCY ANDREASEN   But you still would have given more than
you received, for then you would have gotten up on your—

DENISE LEVERTOV [*laughing*]   On my high horse!

NANCY ANDREASEN   Actually, I was going to say, "on your lec-
ture platform."

ELIZABETH SEWELL   I think the rough times have been the most
valuable because I do think there is a profound cleavage in this
group and it's not that between the literature people and the
medicine people, but between the poets and the academics. I
think it underlies what we've been saying, and that we never
got to it. But perhaps poets and academics shouldn't be gath-
ered under "literature."

JO TRAUTMANN   That division struck me too as I read Denise's
letter, for academics value discourse. Some may call it "hot
air," and occasionally "discourse" is just a euphemism, but
however much we joke about it, it is the way academics grope
towards change and the details of the truth, as Ian has mentioned. We sit down and we reflect together, whether literally
as in this case or figuratively. This is the way we have been
trained to search for the details, and for the most part we like
it. It is a different mode from that normally used by the poet.
Some of us sitting around the table have experience with two
or three different modes of knowing, but I would have thought
that at this table we would give discourse, as I have just described it, a chance, while employing other modes as well.

DENISE LEVERTOV   You know, I've just realized what I've learned
about myself, or rather about myself as a poet—impersonally,
so to speak. That kind of discourse, which for some poets,
including myself, can be very seductive (I like giving my intellect exercise) largely subverts what my poet's instincts need.
Doing this is not good for me as a poet.

JIM COWAN   Because this mode is rationalistic?

DENISE LEVERTOV What I do as a poet is not irrational. However, the focus of energy upon discourse is quite different from the focus of energy in my kind of work.

JO TRAUTMANN Did I hear the hint of a suggestion from Elizabeth that we ought to have left the poets out (though perhaps she meant the academics ought to have been left out)? Should the dialogue group have consisted of medical and literary academics? No, no, I would not like to have left the poets out, to have separated the poets from academics. This *is* a fairly disparate group: we have writers of fiction and writers of poetry among us; we have teachers of writing, teachers of medical students, teachers of literature; we have physicians—a psychiatrist, a pathologist, a surgeon, and an internist; we have administrators too; and I want to say that whatever difficulties we may have had or whatever personal disappointments there may have been, I am very glad we came together.

Are we ready to move on to Denise's paper now? I see that it begins with some of the sentiments she has expressed in the letter.

PAPER FOR LITERATURE AND MEDICINE SYMPOSIUM
Denise Levertov

After attending the "Healing Arts: Literature and Medicine" conferences I find myself no clearer about the subject than I was before the first meeting. Interesting people, and a number of interesting ideas, have been encountered; but a field of thought and endeavor has not—for me at least—been defined. Whatever I thought at the time of receiving the invitation to participate in these symposia, concerning the relationship of the imagination to the capacity for compassion, and concerning the part literature in general (along with the other arts and poetry in particular) might play in stimulating and developing the imagination, I think still; and my views have not been modified in any manner I can discern by the conversations we've had. To make a point of extending to the medical profession a belief in the value of experiencing the arts and humanities, and the opportunity to do so, is to emphasize the obvious. If the experience of literature (while not, as we should humbly remind ourselves, a *sine qua non* for kindness, nor a dependable means to develop it) is potentially a humanizing factor in any life, then of course it must be so for medical students and doctors and nurses as much as for others; and it is equally a matter of course that the medical profession, along with certain others such as social work and schoolteaching, requires the maximum degree of kindness and intelligent empathy from its members. The rationale for introducing more opportunity for study of the arts and humanities into "pre-med" and graduate medical curricula (which I take to be the underlying *raison d'être* of our dialogues, even though we have been encouraged to digress as freely as we desired) surely needs no defense. (Though I have proceeded to make one, as will be seen.)

It might, however, be useful to define further the relationship I have spoken of as existing between the faculties of imagination and compassion. Also of interest might be the way in which the concrete and sensuous experience of language afforded by poetry possibly contributes to a greater awareness, for both speaker and listener—writer and reader—of what is being said and felt in many an interchange of daily "professional" life.

Reading Joanne Trautmann's "Outline for Invited Participants" with which we were presented at the commencement of our meetings, I was struck by the presence of the colon in the general title, which conveys the concept that literature itself is to be regarded as a "healing" art; and also by the phrase, "new attitudes toward the function of literature." These, together with the fact that much of our first meeting was given to debate on what are, to my mind, dubious subjects—"madness and art," "literature and therapy," and so on—gave rise to the statement which follows.

On the Concept of the Arts as Forms of Healing and on "the Function of Literature."

I've written elsewhere about how much I disagree with those who look upon art as pearls produced by sick oysters, and who mistakenly identify the creative and self-destructive impulses which at times coexist in individuals, so I'll not belabor that point afresh. But there is another concept I believe to be equally mistaken: the identification of Art with self-expression.

The logic of this misconception is as follows: (1) Everybody has feelings. (2) Feelings demand expression. (3) Failure to express feelings is akin to constipation—blockage and toxicity of the system results. (4) The means of expressing feeling are common to everyone, and among the most useful are the arts. (5) The arts are not, or should not be, the exclusive possession of an elite. (6) The arts must be enlisted for social use as mild laxatives.

This series is obviously faulty. (1) Yes, everybody has feelings, and (2) feelings demand expression—but they demand expression in the sense of articulation, not of expulsion, of pushing-out-in-order-to-get-rid-of. To articulate is "to utter distinctly," "to set forth in distinct particulars" (that's where its relation to the joints, as of a hand, for instance, becomes clear) "to be systematically interrelated," "to speak so as to be intelligible." To articulate feelings, to make them intelligible, does not involve intellectualizing them out of existence; even less is it a matter of convulsive ejection. The aim is not elimination but absorption. (3) The arts are, indeed, modes of articulation; but though my political standpoint causes me to deplore deliberate, exclusionary elitism, my experience as an artist and as a receiver of art causes me to doubt that the doing of art can be part of everyone's experience; and (4) I certainly object to the commandeering of the arts as utile means of self-expression, for it mistakes the nature of art and takes a part for the whole.

As a receiver of art I know that the articulation of feeling can be experienced vicariously. In experiencing art, we not only are stimulated to empathic realizations, living, let's say, the hopes and fears of a fictive person as we read, even though those hopes and fears do not correspond to actual events in our own lives—for example, one need not be an old man treated harshly by his children to feel with, as well as for, King Lear; we also find in art the expression of our own emotions. We turn to love poems when we are in love, to elegies when we mourn. The gaiety of one song speaks for our own light hearts on a lucky morning, or the sadness of another for our loneliness at a different time. Access to these essential resources must indeed not be confined to an elite; the moral quality of a culture may be judged by their availability.

It is also possible for everyone to partake in some degree in the experience of *using the materials of the arts*, whether the visual or tactile arts; dance; music; theatre; or the writing of poetry or imaginative prose. This experience will be life-enhancing, both in itself and as a means to better reception of works of art made by others; undoubtedly, where therapy is needed, it can be a therapeutic activity—whether or not it is "self-expressive" in the getting-it-off-your-chest, letting-off-steam sense. But, it will not necessarily lead to the creation of works of art.

For while art subsumes in its nature the self-expressive; and is a form of articulation (that is, of setting forth experience, a making intelligible, and so, absorbable, of feelings otherwise unassimilable), it is nevertheless not circumscribed, not to be defined *as* those qualities and those actions. *Art as process* is undertaken by artists (as distinct from persons seeking a means, more or less therapeutic in intent, of self-expression) for its own sake, from an instinctive desire and need to *make*, to form things in a particular medium; and they have towards that medium—be it language, or visual form, or whatsoever—a marked preference not of the intending will but of the sensibility, indeed I would say of the nervous system, which makes them more sensitive not morally or emotionally, but *aesthetically* (at least in regard to their own medium) than others. Even in cultures productive of more popular and anonymous art than our modern Western cultures there are degrees of talent, and the occasional supreme artist stands out above the rest. To the artistic sensibility, process is of intense interest, and though the goal is the finished work, the passion and the pleasure—however much the pleasure may be compounded with struggle and even with pain—is in the making of the work and not in the having finished it. Like God in the book of Genesis, the artist does not wait long in contemplation of what he or she has made, but begins on the next day's work. This presents a contrast to the attitude of the self-expresser, whose satisfaction is typically in the relief of *having expressed*, rather than in the activity of making (which includes self-expression).

David Jones, the British writer and artist, called the artist's work "the gratuitous setting up of altars to the unknown god." Those who utilize the arts for therapeutic purposes often fail to understand this point. They encourage the setting up, in hope of benefit or blessing, of altars to the gods of mental health, self-improvement, or what have you. I don't mean to suggest that the use of poetry, or music, or painting, or any art, as an activity which may help sick people get better or feel happier, is wrong. Two people I know have talked to me very movingly of their work with poetry in such circumstances—one of them working with patients in a psychiatric hospital, one in a rehabilitation program for drug addicts. I also know a number of people, some of them prisoners themselves, who have worked in jails teaching writing and painting. I appreciate the value and importance of such programs (and sometimes buried talent can emerge in them). They can make all the difference to people whose lives are grim and hopeless.

Writing or painting is not going to solve the problems that put people in mental hospitals or in jails, nor keep the terminal cancer patient from death; but it can help people grow, and to feel better about themselves because they are *articulating* in some way; and to live more fully, as long as they *are* alive, than they would have done if they had not written or painted. All that is incontrovertibly good. What is not good is that those who introduce these possibilities (especially to those who are not dying and are not even shut up in institutions) frequently fail to make any distinction between the activities they promote and art itself. The same is true in schools and colleges, in thousands of creative writing workshops. The manipulation of materials and the relief experienced through articulation, though both are factors in the making of works of art, are only factors and not the thing itself; it is misleading to let students suppose they are doing art when in fact they are only taking steps toward doing so. Unless they have that natural, unteachable bent toward a particular medium, and that instinctive drive to make autonomous things, those steps will lead them only to a subjective, private, and temporary satisfaction, not without value, but lower in the scale of possible human experience than it is claimed to be.

I have been speaking of art as process. What of works of art after the process, what of the reception of art as it affects the self? I believe fervently in the role of the arts as essential nourishment for human beings in good health, and therefore must conclude that they can be potent as therapy likewise. The imagination, the aesthetic sense, the capacity for sensuous pleasure, can atrophy like anything else not used, starve if not fed. And these faculties interact with the emotions and so with moral sensitivity: compassion, as I've said elsewhere, is a function of the imagination. But discriminating intelligence is an essential factor in receptivity to art; without it, a mere appetite can devour shoddy substitutes for real literature (or any other art) just as the body's appetite, in ignorance and habitually ill-fed, can fail to recognize the worthlessness and actual harmfulness of soggy white bread and franks full of nitrates and nitrites, followed by flavored sugar, and thinks it has had a nourishing meal. And the emphasis on self-expression in process can affect discrimination in reception—or consumption, to follow through the analogy.

The presentation to students (including patients in therapeutic programs) of masses of inferior literature merely for the sake of supposed relevancy is a part of the same problem. The "relevant" in reading material is closely equivalent to the "self-expressive" in writing. I'm not saying it makes sense to present highly complex works in archaic English to barely literate students of narrow experience, for instance; merely that though there can be found work which is both comprehensible and of high quality, too often familiarity of scene or subject is made the standard of relevancy, in an extension of the principle of self-expressive process: identify, establish previous acquaintance, and proceed to *spew forth*. "Identify" as I'm using it here has both its meanings: In a self-expressive act, the person's own emotions are identified; in a receptive act, what is described is identified *with*. Both are useful, necessary, affirmative in potential. The trouble lies in assuming them to be ends, not means; or rather, that they are assumed to be means for attaining elimination instead of absorption and transformation.

Transformation! Yes, that is probably the key word. *To spew forth* is not to transform; neither is *to state*. Both can be included in the process of making a work of art. But works of art transcend these and other factors, *transforming* them, along with the raw material of experience (factual or emotional) into autonomous creations that give off mysterious energy. Not everyone has the form-sense and the impulse to *make things out of a particular medium* that distinguish the artist; therefore not everyone can effect transformation of raw material (and most artists in one medium—say language—cannot effect transformation in another, such as paint or clay). Nevertheless, everyone has the potential (however undeveloped) to experience works of art created by others, and partake of that transforming communion.

What does the non-artist working in an art medium experience that is of value, then? I think he can experience deeper self-understanding, clarifying articulation, and emotional release. Surely he does not have to be deceived into supposing he is creating works of art in order to experience those benefits. When the non-artist is so deceived, his ability to receive the transforming power of actual works of art is adversely affected because he is not able to distinguish the shoddy from the authentic. If in his own writing or painting he learns no structural and aesthetic standards, but instead evaluates what he and his peers do purely on a basis of how "self-expressive" it is, how can he develop the ability to respond to the great works which would give him the deepest, most transforming, powerfully enlivening experience? Instinct and intuition can be warped, diverted, corrupted. When this happens, the non-artist probably will turn for succor to the substandard, for its very familiarity.

The great power of art is to transform, renovate, activate. If there is a relationship between art and healing it is that. But its power cannot manifest itself if the arts are pressed into servitude and reduced to mere means to an end. The more clearly the self-expressive is defined as usefully that and no more, and the less confusion there is between expulsion and transformative absorption, the more can art act in human lives, making them fuller, more active, more human.

Certainly if one accepts this concept of the essentially affirmative nature of art, then at least one of the topics to which our attention has been addressed, that of "Madness and Art," can be seen as a side-issue at best, while "Art and Health" (or "Literature and Health") would seem to have been a more relevant issue.

Searching for a way to engage myself usefully with our task (or rather, to define for myself what, indeed, our task has been), I tried again to examine the prickly question of whether poetry might have a special, particular relevance for the medical profession. By "poetry" I mean the language of poetry—language as poetry reveals it.

But why for doctors more than for sociologists or urban planners or agronomists? I believe that whatever can detract the scientifically-oriented mind from tendencies to detach words and ideas from their roots in feeling and image is to the good. But is it necessary to keep reiterating this point? Perhaps. Perhaps it is necessary, for even here in our group—brilliant, concerned, and literate though its members are—have we not heard and read considerable quantities of abstraction? When Emerson said that language was "fossil poetry" he meant to remind us that even words seemingly created to expressly convey abstractions still embody concrete images. This is what intellect forgets or denies whenever it is too exclusively cultivated, to the neglect of the sensuous, aesthetic, emotional, or instinctive elements.

The unthinking use of "negative and positive" is a curious case and one that is unfortunately too well-established to admit of revision. Doctor and patient are relieved when a test proves "negative"; both are sorry when it is "positive" (though I cannot help supposing that many a diagnostician with a hunch has been more gratified—for a moment, at least—at finding his guess was correct than distressed at the implication for his patient: if, that is, he is one of those physicians whose ability to empathize is stunted). And take the word *patient.* How many doctors stop to reflect upon the nuances of that word—nuances relating to endurance, passivity, subjection to the actions of others, pain and forebearance?

Because it is more condensed, poetry, even more than good prose, depends for its very life on an awareness of these root meanings. It is not poetry's only vital organ, this awareness, any more than the heart or the liver is a human body's sole vital organ. Nevertheless, like them, it is genuinely indispensable. When I speak of awareness I do not mean that the poet is necessarily constantly conscious of etymology, or that he or she need to have made a special study of it; rather I mean that the poet's feeling for language must provide an acute sensitivity to verbal interconnections, and enough concern to investigate and verify the history of relationships intuited by the ear.

How does this affect the reader? Again, not necessarily by demanding of him or her a consciousness of every nuance, but rather a receptiveness to the effects brought about through the writer's awareness, open to the total experience. Yet the attentive reading of poetry habituates the reader to a precise, concrete, sensuous employment of language, so that when sloppy, ineffective, lifeless language is encountered it is less likely to be tolerated. For example, the redundancies mentioned by Ian Lawson in his paper "The Place of Language in Medical Science and Practice" and in his quoted article, "The Language of Geriatric Care," are even less tolerable to a reader used to the concise precisions of poetry than they would be to the reader accustomed to good prose. Ian's professional objection to the proliferations of nomenclature is on "practical" grounds; mine would be "aesthetic." I do see a practical consideration in my aesthetics— namely that lifeless language simply does not function with full power even in the most routine ways. To put it another way, it tends to make actions routine that should be continually refreshed: actions such as nursing procedures. It is in such considerations that one may perhaps see a relationship between the more demanding and sophisticated "ear" developed by the study of poetry, and ethics. Beyond the value it can have for *any* person or category of persons, poetry can have, for those whose attention is apt to be intensely focused on a narrow or discrete area, a special usefulness, stimulating the imagination as it does, revealing analogies, and, by its concrete, sensuous, image-rooted vocabulary, redirecting the sensibility to the underlying dynamics of language.

For a doctor this greater sensitivity to language might well mean the development of a keener ear for the emotions and sensations which patients, however restricted their means of articulation, might be trying to express. (It may here be of interest to note, by the way, that in Britain, where medical care has become increasingly dependent on doctors to whom English is a second language, and whose knowledge of idiomatic and regional speech patterns is scanty, special dictionaries and phrase-books have been prepared. This has been done so that the doctor will know what the patient means when he says he "feels woozy and his earlug hurts.")

By the same token, a language-sensitive physician might be enabled, by careful and imaginative word-choice, to impart more efficiently to patients and their families, and also to nurses and other co-workers, information they need to know. The same holds true, of course, for nurses themselves and other medical personnel. This more accurate and flexible comprehension and utilization of language is not separable from the awakened and functioning imagination. Empathy and compassion, functions of the imagination, lead to the "inspired" word or phrase, the verbal accuracy which leads to further enlightenment, and in turn to a deeper comprehension of the situation.[3]

Of the topics Denise raised and the group pursued, the one most central to the basic thesis—that literature and medicine can both be healing arts—was initially rephrased by Elizabeth Sewell, who noted the "enormously interesting circle of health, nourishment, and energy" in the paper, as these qualities were released by art. Elizabeth wanted to affirm that "an active involvement" with art, whether as doer or receiver, was a part of good health. Denise continued, stating that health was "fullness of being," and that she could scarcely imagine calling someone healthy who beyond physical health was not also healthy in that part of the self which is nourished by art. In response, Elizabeth seemed to take a few steps more when she declined to separate mind (or "soul" or "personality") in this respect from body, evincing again her tendency towards synthesis. At one point she told the group she wanted to consider whether or not we humans had the potential for imagining ourselves or dreaming ourselves into total health of the body-mind, this power to be released by art, a suggestion she had broached as early as the first meeting.

Heretofore, the dialogists had for the most part spoken of literature as a healing art on the level of its helping us to perceive matters more clearly or to imagine them more compassionately. Ian Lawson reiterated this point as Denise's paper was being discussed with the statement that "literature gives patients a voice for their suffering." But Elizabeth had urged herself, at least, towards another level entirely—a level on which literature becomes more directly a health giver, and Emerson's remark about the only true doctor being the poet, a literal description of professional skills.

Bill Ober attempted to clarify positions by asking both Denise and Elizabeth whether literature was indispensable for good health or whether it could be done away with, like the spleen. The dialogists hedged in reply, their inference being that the answer lay in the area of faith or hope. At first no one wanted to take on the pathologist, who obviously was looking for fact. Then Dick Selzer told this little story:

"I made a small sociological survey of my own. We have a summer cottage by the shore near New Haven. It is in a decidedly working-class area, and the men and women that I encounter during my free time in the summer are my neighbors there. Please do not think I am, in describing them this way, saying anything pejorative about them. I love them. One is a maintenance man. Most of them are factory workers or people who work in the sanitation department.

"When I first began to go there, I wanted to make friends with these people. I wanted this very much; I found their laughter infectious. But gradually I began to find myself very restless. I felt that I was constructing a false premise upon which we were to be friends. In fact, I was bored. So I decided to look around for whatever creative thing, whatever art, in its broadest sense, they pursued, and then I would orient myself in that direction, even if it were gardening or growing bonsai or carving wood. I cold-bloodedly began to hunt and peck around the neighborhood for art. But the same thing happened every night—we sat on the stoop and drank beer. They complained about their jobs. They were bored stiff with each other, with themselves, and with me. I couldn't find the artistic spirit of these people. They were a consumer group who were angry because they didn't have enough money (actually they did), whose total thought processes had to do with conniving at the little details of putting one over on the boss.

"In the end, I took a great risk. Denise, I always remember the story you told about your mother's childhood in Wales, when the men would squat outside their houses and sing. Even though each was singing separately, the voices would mingle in this town. It is such a beautiful idea. Well, I decided one day this summer to gather my neighbors together on my stoop. And I said, 'I'm going to read you a story.' This shocked and amazed everybody. I heard my middle son say to my older son, 'He's going to make an ass of himself.'

"But I was determined to do this thing. I chose a story called 'The Only Good Indian,' and the reason I chose it, in fact wrote it at that time, was to answer the racist who delights in the weaknesses of other ethnic groups. Although the story has a racist title, it turns out that the only good person is the Indian. The story had to do with the Mohawk Indians who are very good at doing the super structures of high bridges, but since we introduced them to fire water, some drink too much, and during the course of building the Quinnipiac River Bridge, one of them fell from the super structure into a piling of wet concrete, and therefore was unable to be found—ever. The point was, they should have named the bridge after him.

"I read this dynamite of a story to these guys with all the power that I had, and by the time I had finished, half of them had left and the other half were so embarrassed for me they could have died. It was a total failure. I just gave up. I said, 'Where is it?' And I never want to go back. Not because all the women wear those pink plastic curlers in their hair—I don't feel superior to them—but I just want to find out what it is that feeds their spirit."

Here Dick hesitated, and several of the dialogists, but chiefly Denise, stated for him what seemed the obvious conclusion: his neighbors were unhealthy and the tale an illustration of the thesis that without an active involvement with art, all people are unhealthy. Nevertheless, Dick himself gave the moral of the story in the form of a sighing answer to Bill Ober's question: "No, art is not indispensable for health." His neighbors were healthy, and they had certainly dispensed with him.

Mary Stephens, one of the Institute's liaison representatives, gave a different perspective. She said that the dialogue had "deepened and enriched [her] belief in the oneness of things," and reminded the group that earlier civilizations, as well as some contemporary ones, would have assumed the unity of health and art. "How is it," she asked, "that in our particular culture the physician as healer and the artist as healer have diverged so greatly over the past centuries?" Mary went on to suggest that myth might be worth exploring as an area which unifies story and practice. Her brief presentation took the group from Jessie Weston's discussion of "The Medicine Man"[4] (who within himself fuses the functions of literature, medicine, and religion), through the health-giving aspects of the stories of Jesus and Sir Gawain, back to the catharsis of Greek tragedy, and finally to Apollo—the god of truth, music, and health.

18 September 1976
Inevitably, the discussion at the last session centered around the future of literature and medicine. Each dialogist presented some topics for further investigation or suggestions for specific action. On reflection, the items seemed linked to each person's view of what had happened during the meetings and to the manner in which he or she had participated.

For instance, Nancy Andreasen, who was one of the most astute observers of the ways in which the group interacted, thought she might undertake "an examination of the impact of drama based in part on what psychiatrists and psychologists have come to know about the process of group dynamics." She wondered if "a play which draws on this process is a better one, that is, more powerful."

Jim Cowan mentioned "the history of science, and medicine in particular, and the parallel history of literature and criticism." Realizing the scope of such a topic as stated, Jim offered two very specialized sub-topics: "Medicine, the New Science, and John Donne" and "The Humours and Renaissance Comedy." In the latter topic, Jim implied that the approach would be similar to the one Bill Ober had taken in his paper on the eighteenth-century spleen. Jim thought a course could be developed which would enable medical students to study the histories of medicine and literature together in a "history of ideas" format.

Ian Lawson spoke in terms of "divergent and convergent topics" for further interdisciplinary discussion, and obviously enjoyed the prospect of doing both. As an example of a convergent topic he offered "love of language and language skills in medical writing and creativity"; as a divergent, "further work-out on the nature of objectivity."

Denise Levertov objected to divergent topics, or at least to their discussion by groups such as this one. Neither side, she declared, convinced the other, so it was as if no one had spoken at all. She found such conversation "irritatingly banal." Instead, Denise urged writers to act. She referred to the "need for us to witness sickness and death and social trouble, even if we have to seek it out, as in Wiseman's films."[5] She thought writers could interview patients better than sociologists could. When asked by Nancy Andreasen to defend that statement, Denise said that "writers could punctuate their transcriptions right!"

Gene Moss revealed his receptiveness to some of Elizabeth Sewell's ideas, his plans for further reading in clinical medicine, and his firm commitment to the healing arts through his suggestion of " 'stress' and its management by the human imagination" as a possibility for the future.

Bill Ober argued for more education and research, including a journal of medicine and literature,[6] an annual workshop conducted by the Humanities Department of Penn State's College of Medicine for teachers of both medical and literary students, and a dual degree program leading to the M.D. and the Ph.D. in English.

Dick Selzer had highly personal plans. He wanted to think about "man's habitat from the standpoint of literature, including the body and the earth and the interface between them." He refined the subject to mean "the body as a dwelling-place *and* inhabitant." Included in his list of things to read were the novels of doctor-writer Walker Percy.

Elizabeth Sewell posed her topics as "questions"—as in "the question of death" and "the question of isolation and passivity (the helpless feeling, not cooperation) experienced by patients in hospitals." Although she made no specific reference to literature here, Elizabeth implied that the alert writer and teacher of literature might responsibly have a very broad role indeed.

Jo Trautmann set herself several assignments in literature and

medicine, chiefly the shaping of these meetings for anyone interested in reading about them. It would be difficult to separate
the personalities from the concepts, and the concepts from the
process. She decided to take the dialogue—which had been by
turns perceptive, glib, banal, profound, angering, astonishing,
moving, hilarious, frustrating, self-seeking, and outward-reach-
ing—and attempt to demonstrate how much the dialogists had
discovered as well as how they came to do it.

Notes
Index

Notes

FOREWORD

1. John Henry Newman. Inaugural Address to the Faculty of Arts, Catholic University of Ireland, 1854.

2. In addition to this book, the other publications in this series are: *Nourishing the Humanistic in Medicine: Interactions with the Social Sciences*, William R. Rogers and David Barnard, eds. (Pittsburgh: University of Pittsburgh Press, 1979); *Medicine and Religion: Strategies of Care*, Donald W. Shriver, Jr., ed. (Pittsburgh: University of Pittsburgh Press, 1980); and a manuscript on the fine arts edited by Geri Berg, which is scheduled for publication in 1982 from Southern Illinois University Press.

PROLOGUE

1. Since this dialogue took place, two useful publications have become available. See the anthology of primary materials: Joseph Ceccio, *Medicine in Literature* (New York: Longman Press, 1978); and a collection of critical essays: Enid Rhodes Peschel, ed., *Medicine and Literature* (New York: Neale Watson Academic Publications, Inc., 1980).

MEETING ONE

1. Nancy Andreasen, "Ariel's Flight: The Death of Sylvia Plath," *Journal of the American Medical Association*, 288 (1974): 595–9.

2. Jo Trautmann had suggested six topics to get the group started. In addition to the two mentioned by Denise Levertov, the other topics were: the doctor as mythic figure; irrationality in medicine; medicine and art as central visions in the twentieth century; and the doctor as writer.

165

3. Arthur C. Clarke, *Profiles of the Future* (New York: Harper & Row, 1962).

4. Bruno Bettelheim, *The Informed Heart* (Glencoe, Ill.: The Free Press, 1960), p. 261.

5. The play (1973) by Peter Shaffer.

6. Carl R. Rogers, "The Necessary and Sufficient Conditions of Therapeutic Personality Change," *Journal of Consulting Psychology*, 21 (1957): 95–103.

7. James Kirkup, "A Correct Compassion. To Mr. Philip Allison, after watching him perform a Mitral Valvulotomy in the General Infirmary at Leeds," in *A Correct Compassion and Other Poems* (London: Oxford University Press, 1952).

8. For instance, A. R. Feinstein, "Taxonomy and Logic in Clinical Data," *Annals of the New York Academy of Science*, 161 (1969): 450–9; and by the same author, *Clinical Judgment* (Huntington, New York: R. E. Krieger Publishing Co., 1967).

9. Francis Walshe, "The Nature and Dimensions of Nosography in Modern Medicine," *The Lancet*, CCLXXI (1956), 6952:1060–3.

10. Lawrence L. Weed, *Medical Records, Medical Education, and Patient Care* (Cleveland: The Press of Case Western Reserve University, 1970).

11. E. Fuller Torrey, *The Mind Game: Witch Doctors and Psychiatrists* (New York: Emerson Hall, 1972).

12. The participants decided that fairly comprehensive answers to these practical questions are attempted by Joanne Trautmann in her syllabi for the literature courses taught to medical students at Penn State College of Medicine and her book, written with Carol Pollard, *Literature and Medicine: Topics, Titles and Notes* (Philadelphia: Society for Health and Human Values, 1975), and University of Pittsburgh Press, 1982.

MEETING TWO

1. Denise Levertov, "Anne Sexton: Light up the Cave," *Ramparts* (December 1974 / January 1975), pp. 61–63.

2. That essay was too long to be included here, but William B. Ober's methodology, as well as a good deal of information about literature and

medicine, may be found in his *Boswell's Clap and Other Essays* (Carbondale, Ill.: Southern Illinois University Press, 1979).

3. Cesare Lombroso, *The Man of Genius* (London: Walter Scott, 1891).

4. W. Lange-Eichbaum, *The Problem of Genius* (London: Kegan Paul, 1931); J. F. Nisbet, *The Insanity of Genius* (London: Grant Richards, 1900); T. B. Hyslop, *The Great Abnormals* (New York: George H. Doran, 1925).

5. J. L. Karlsson, "Genetic Association of Giftedness and Creativity with Schizophrenia," *Hereditas* 66 (1970): 177–82; T. F. McNeill, "Prebirth and Postbirth Influence on the Relationship Between Creative Ability and Recorded Mental Illness," *Journal of Personality* 39 (1971): 391–406; A. Juda, "The Relationship Between Highest Mental Capacity and Psychic Abnormalities," *American Journal of Psychiatry* 106 (1949): 296–307; H. A. Ellis, *A Study of British Genius* (New York: Houghton Mifflin, 1926).

6. N. J. C. Andreasen and A. Canter, "The Creative Writer: Psychiatric Symptoms and Family History in Creative Writers," *Life History Research in Psychopathology*, vol. 4, G. Wirt, G. Winokur, and M. Roth, eds. (Minneapolis: University of Minnesota Press, 1975), pp. 187–210.

7. This essay has been printed as "The Surgeon as Priest," in Richard Selzen *Mortal Lessons* (New York: Simon and Schuster, 1976).

8. Lawrence's works are cited parenthetically in my text by abbreviated title and page numbers as follows:

CP	*The Complete Poems of D. H. Lawrence*, ed. Vivian de Sola Pinto and Warren Roberts (New York: Viking, 1971).
EP	*Etruscan Places* (New York: Viking, Compass, 1968).
FU	*Fantasia of the Unconscious*, in *Psychoanalysis and the Unconscious and Fantasia of the Unconscious* (New York: Viking, Compass, 1960).
K	*Kangaroo* (Melbourne, London, Toronto: Heinemann, 1955).
LCL	*Lady Chatterley's Lover* (New York: Grove, 1959).
MEH	*Movements in European History* (Oxford: Oxford University Press, Humphrey Milford, 1925).
MWD	*St. Mawr and The Man Who Died* (New York: Vintage Books, n.d.).
P	*Phoenix: The Posthumous Papers of D. H. Lawrence*,

ed. Edward D. McDonald (New York: Viking, 1968).

P II   *Phoenix II: Uncollected, Unpublished, and Other
        Prose Works by D. H. Lawrence*, ed. Warren Roberts
        and Harry T. Moore (New York: Viking, 1968).

PU   *Psychoanalysis and the Unconscious*, in *Psycho-
        analysis and the Unconscious and Fantasia of the
        Unconscious* (New York: Viking, Compass, 1960).

9. See T. S. Eliot, *The Complete Poems and Plays, 1909–1950* (New York: Harcourt, 1958), p. 3.

10. See Stephen Spender, "D. H. Lawrence" (audio-tape) (Cincinnati: Sound Seminars, McGraw-Hill 75910, n.d.).

11. See Kate Millett, *Sexual Politics* (Garden City, N.Y.: Doubleday, 1970), pp. 240, 243–44.

MEETING THREE

1. A. R. Feinstein, *Clinical Judgment* (Huntington, N.Y.: R. E. Krieger Publishing Co., 1967), p. 13.

2. Kenneth Burke, *A Grammar of Motives* (Berkeley: University of California Press, 1969), pp. xviii–xix.

3. Lewis Thomas, *The Lives of a Cell: Notes of a Biology Watcher* (New York: Viking Press, 1974), pp. 94–95.

4. "A Taxonomy of Geriatric Care Using the Problem-Oriented Record System," in *The Language of Geriatric Care: Implications for Professional Review*, Ian R. Lawson and Stanley R. Ingman, eds. Connecticut Health Research Series, No. 6, 1975, pp. 26–27.

5. Stafford Beer, *Platform for Change* (London: John Wiley & Sons, 1975), pp. 170–71.

6. Denise Levertov, *Life in the Forest* (New York: New Directions, 1978). "Artist to Intellectual (Poet to Explainer)" is reproduced here with the first and third sections interchanged.

7. In a fragment from an unpublished manuscript of Coleridge's, quoted in Alice D. Snyder, *Coleridge on Logic and Learning* (New Haven: Yale University Press, 1929), app. B.

8. At the previous day's meeting, Dick Selzer had told the group of his recent experience at an abortion. Eventually his observations were published as "What I saw at the Abortion," *Esquire*, January 1976, pp.

66–67; and reprinted as "Abortion" in his *Mortal Lessons* (New York: Simon and Schuster, 1976).

9. William Faulkner, *As I Lay Dying* in *The Sound and the Fury* and *As I Lay Dying* (New York: Random House, Modern Library, 1946), p. 510.

MEETING FOUR

1. Joanne Trautmann, "William Carlos Williams and the Poetry of Medicine," *Ethics in Science and Medicine* 2 (1975): 105–14.

2. The incident Joanne Trautmann relates here became the basis for Richard Selzer's story, "Amazons," published in Richard Selzer, *Confessions of a Knife* (New York: Simon and Schuster, 1979).

3. A. Alvarez, *The Savage God* (New York: Random House, 1972).

4. For instance, see Nancy Y. Hoffman, "The Doctor as Scapegoat: A Study in Ambivalence," *Journal of the American Medical Association* 220 (1972): 58–61.

5. Published as "Abortion," in Richard Selzer, *Mortal Lessons* (New York: Simon and Schuster, 1976).

6. *The Island* hasn't received much critical attention. But Ronald Hingley, in his *A New Life of Anton Chekhov* (New York: Knopf, 1976), considers the book of great importance and devotes about twenty pages to it. "What possessed Chekhov to undertake this bizarre expedition?" Hingley asks. "He has explained his reasons frankly, repetitively and at length in his letters of early 1890; but the more closely we scrutinize this material the less does any single, overriding purpose emerge" (p. 128).

7. *The Island*, trans. Luba and Michael Terpak (New York: Washington Square Press, 1967), p. xxxiii.

8. All Chekhov's letters are quoted from the selected edition by Avrahm Yarmolinsky (New York: Viking Press, 1973).

MEETING FIVE

1. This quotation is from a letter written by Joanne Trautmann, asking each dialogist to list the topics not covered in our meetings, but of potential interest to the group.

2. The social sciences dialogue was published as *Nourishing the Hu-*

manistic in Medicine: Interactions with the Social Sciences, William R. Rogers and David Bernard, eds. (Pittsburgh: University of Pittsburgh Press, 1979).

3. The rest of Denise Levertov's paper, omitted here, dealt with two other subjects proposed by Joanne Trautmann at the beginning of the meetings—Responsibility to the Self versus Responsibility to the Community and The Nature of Objectivity.

4. Jessie L. Weston, *From Ritual to Romance* (New York: Doubleday, 1957), chap. 8 (originally published in 1920).

5. Frederick Wiseman's documentary films, such as *Hospital* and *Titicut Follies*.

6. The *Literature and Medicine Review* has been launched by Kathryn A. Rabuzzi of the Department of English at Syracuse University.

Index

Index

Index

Elizabeth I (queen of England), 90
Ellis, Havelock, 32, 167 n.5
Emerson, Ralph Waldo, 154; "The Poet," 2
empathy, 17; in medicine, 13, 55; through literature, 149–50
Empedocles, 85, 87
End of the World, The" (MacLeish), 118–19
Energy: and health, 8, 156
Epidauros (Greece), 45–46, 70, 87
Equus (Shaffer), 16, 166 n.5
Etruscan Places (Lawrence), 59–60
eudemony: as device for evaluating medicine, 76

Fall of the House of Usher, The (Poe), 116
Fantasia of the Unconscious (Lawrence), 60–63, 69, 141
Faulkner, William: As I Lay Dying, 99
Faust: in Goethe, 87
fear: in medicine, 77
Feinstein, Alvan, 18, 73, 166 n.8, 168 n.1
femininity: in Lawrence, 57, 64–65
Ficino, Marsilio, 85
Ford, Gerald, 15
Freud, Sigmund, 28
Frost, Robert, 26

Gawain, Sir, 159
Geber, 85
genetic research, 11
geriatrics, 75
Gnostic texts, 86
Goethe, Johann von, 85; Faust, 87
"Gooseberries" (Chekhov), 131–32, 135
Gordon, Burgess, 74
Gray, Thomas: "The Bard," 112
Gray's Anatomy of the Human Body, 61–62, 69
guilt: doctors' feelings of, 14–16
"Gusev" (Chekhov), 136–37

Hamlet (Shakespeare), 30–31, 116
handicaps, 66
Hardy, Thomas, 117

Harper, George Mills, 86
Health: definition of, 8, 20–21, 156. See also Imagination, in health and illness; Sanity
Heisenberg uncertainty principle, 76
Heller, Joseph, 117
Hemingway, Ernest, 117
Hermes (Trismegistus), 85
Hippolytus, 29
Hopkins, Gerard Manley, 116
Horace, 117
Human Sexual Inadequacy (Masters and Johnson), 66
Human Sexual Response (Masters and Johnson), 65–66
Humours, the, 159
Hypnosis: definition and relation to magic of, 108–9

Iamblichus, 85
Illness, 54–55, 160. See also Depression; Imagination, in health and illness; Schizophrenia
Imagination: atrophy of, 152; compassion's relation to, 12, 152; dangers of, 106; in health and illness, 87–88, 104–5, 108, 109, 130–32, 156–59, 160; inaccessible to rationality, 80–81; method of, 86–87, 90, 92; role of, in assessing patients, 77; role of, in dying, 111
Insanity. See Madness
Institute on Human Values in Medicine, xv, xvi, 143
Internal medicine, 52
International Classification of Disease, 18
"In the Cart" (Chekhov), 132
Intuition, 53–54, 57
Iowa, University of, Writers' Workshop, 32–33, 34–35
Island: A Journey to Sakhalin, The (Chekhov), 127–35

JAMA (Journal of the American Medical Association), 5, 165 n.1
Jesus: as healer and scapegoat, 107, 159
Joachim of Flora, 57
Job, 29

173

Index

Johnson, Samuel, 33; *Rasselas*, 112
Jones, David, 150–51
Joyce, James, 26, 117; *Dubliners*, 133; *A Portrait of the Artist as a Young Man*, 63
"Jubilate Agno" (Smart), 119
Juda, Adele, 32, 167 n.5
Judgment: in clinical practice, 73
Juvenal, 117

Kafka, Franz: "A Country Doctor," 134
Kangaroo (Lawrence), 57–58
Kant, Immanuel, 102
Keats, John, 33, 51
Kirkup, James: *Correct Compassion*, 17
Kraepelin, Emil, 28
"Kubla Khan" (Coleridge), 112, 119–22

Lady Chatterley's Lover (Lawrence), 55, 63–66, 70
Langer, Susanne K., 94
Language: analogous to anatomy, 9; barrier to understanding magic, 110; and the computer, 73; explosion medicine, 74–75; "fossil poetry," 154; identifies ambiguity, 72; matrix of thought and action in medicine, 72–73; and measurement, 94; methods of, 7; in modern medical care, 17–20; as nonsense, 118–19; as rational medium in art, 114; sensitivity to, valuable for doctors, 154–56
Lawrence, D. H., 12, 20, 55–70, 94, 98. Works cited: "Chastity," 58–59; *Etruscan Places*, 59–60; *Fantasia of the Unconscious*, 60–63, 69, 141; *Kangaroo*, 57–58; *Lady Chatterley's Lover*, 55, 63–66, 70; *The Man Who Died*, 66–69; *Movements in European History*, 57; "Noli Me Tangere," 58; *Pansies*, 58–59; *Psychoanalysis and the Unconscious*, 60, 69, 142; Review of Leo Tolstoi's *Resurrection*, 56; "The Risen Lord," 56; *St. Mawr*, 97; "Snake," 95; *Sons and Lovers*, 67; "Sun in Me," 56; "Touch," 58

Lawson, Ian, 96, 155; as dialogist, 17–19, 51, 52, 54–55, 70, 77, 89, 93, 144–45, 156–57, 159–60; paper by, 71–77; sketch of, xvii
Leibnitz, Gottfried, 85
Levertov, Denise, 23, 71, 97, 125, 166 n.1; as dialogist, 1, 2, 3, 4, 5–6, 9, 10, 12–13, 14, 16, 17, 20, 50, 53, 54, 77, 79, 89, 90, 91, 93, 140, 141, 142–43, 146, 147, 156, 158, 160; letter from, 138–39; paper by, 147–56; poem by, 78–79; sketch of, xvii
Life Studies (Lowell), 25–26
Literary criticism, 51, 97–98
Literary research: value of, 1–2
Literature: rewards of teaching, 2; as therapy, 5–6, 149–53; value of teaching, 4; value of, for medical people, 12, 14 passim. See also Drama; Poetry
Literature academics: their use of language, 1
Lombroso, Cesare, 32, 166 n.3
"London" (Blake), 117–18
Lourdes (France), 43
Love: and healing, 48, 70; as "non-possessive warmth," 17; surgery as, 40
"Love Song of J. Alfred Prufrock, The" (Eliot), 55–56
Low, Barbara, 61
Lowell, Robert, 23, 27; *Life Studies*, 25–26; "Waking in the Blue," 26

McElhinney, Thomas, xvi
MacLean (Hospital), 26
MacLeish, Archibald: "Ars Poetica," 97; "The End of the World," 118–19
Madness, 20; in the artist, 111–12; artistic patterns in, 112–13; in Chekhov, 129, 131–35; and creativity, 23–24, 32–36; danger of, with Apollo, 106–7; definition of, 99; akin to ecstasy, 116, 119–22; in literature, 113–23; as method of study, 92; as reflection of romantic values, 23, 31–32, 111–12; in satire, 117–18
Magic: implications for medicine of,

Index

Index

TABLE DES MATIÈRES

ACHEVÉ D'IMPRIMER
SUR LES PRESSES DE
L'IMPRIMERIE DES REMPARTS S.A.
À YVERDON
POUR LES
ÉDITIONS DE LA BACONNIÈRE
À NEUCHÂTEL (SUISSE)
LE 30 AVRIL 1980